Dora Feest

Breakfast
FOR A Better Body

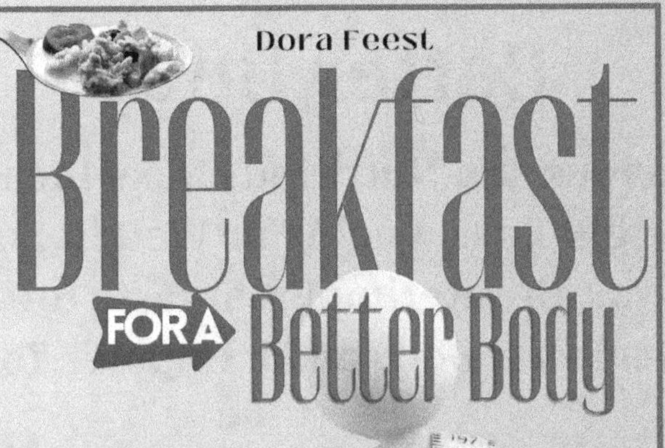

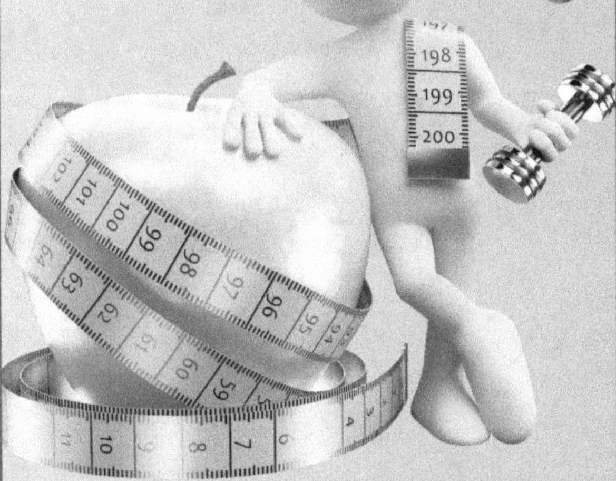

DELICIOUS AND NUTRITIOUS MEAL IDEAS FOR WEIGHT LOSS

FUEL YOUR WEIGHT LOSS: MOUTHWATERING BREAKFASTS FOR A HEALTHIER BODY AND A HAPPIER YOU!

Breakfast for a Better Body

Delicious and Nutritious Meal Ideas for Weight Loss. Fuel Your Weight Loss: Mouthwatering Breakfasts for a Healthier Body and a Happier You!

Written by:

Dora Feest

Content:

Introduction

Chapter 1: The Breakfast Revolution: Unleashing the Power of a Nutritious Morning Meal

Chapter 4: From the Grains to Glory: Wholesome Cereal and Oatmeal Delights

Creative and nutritious cereal and oatmeal recipes

Incorporate a range of grains to add diversity and maximize nutritional value

Choose whole grains and avoiding added sugars in packaged cereals for optimal nutrition

Chapter 5: Egg-Cellent Creations: Protein-Packed Breakfasts

Egg-based recipes for protein-rich breakfasts

Vegetarian alternatives using tofu or legumes

Incorporating vegetables and herbs for added flavor and nutrients

Chapter 8: The Science of Weight Loss: How Food Affects Your Body and Mind

Conclusion

INTRODUCTION

The Importance of Breakfast for Weight Loss and Overall Health.

Breakfast is often hailed as the most important meal of the day, and for good reason. Whether you're aiming to lose weight or simply improve your overall health, starting your morning with a nutritious breakfast can have a profound impact on your well-being.

When it comes to weight loss, breakfast plays a crucial role in jumpstarting your metabolism. After a night of fasting, your body's metabolic rate tends to be lower, and eating breakfast helps rev up your engine. By providing your body with essential nutrients early in the day, you kickstart your metabolism, allowing it to efficiently burn calories throughout the day.

Skipping breakfast, on the other hand, can have detrimental effects on weight loss efforts. Research shows that individuals who skip breakfast are more likely to overeat later in the day, leading to excessive calorie intake and potential weight gain. Additionally, prolonged fasting can slow down metabolism and make it harder to shed pounds.

A well-balanced breakfast not only aids in weight loss but also provides numerous health benefits. It sets the stage for healthier food choices throughout the day, as starting off with a nutritious meal helps regulate appetite and reduces cravings for unhealthy snacks. By fueling your body with the right nutrients in the morning, you're more likely to make mindful choices when it comes to your other meals. Furthermore, a nutritious breakfast provides sustained energy that supports physical and mental performance. It replenishes glycogen stores, the primary fuel source for your brain and muscles, allowing you to stay focused, alert, and productive throughout the day. This can enhance your exercise performance and overall productivity, positively impacting both your weight loss journey and daily life.

Incorporating a variety of nutrients into your breakfast is key to reaping its benefits. Including lean protein, high-fiber carbohydrates, and healthy fats ensures a balanced meal that keeps you satiated and prevents energy crashes. This combination promotes stable blood sugar levels, preventing excessive hunger and overeating later in the day.

Moreover, breakfast provides an excellent opportunity to meet your daily nutritional needs. By including nutrient-dense foods like fruits, vegetables, whole grains, and lean proteins, you can pack your breakfast with vitamins, minerals, antioxidants, and essential macronutrients. These nutrients not only support weight loss but also bolster your immune system, improve digestion, and contribute to overall well-being.

In conclusion, breakfast is a vital component of a successful weight loss journey and a healthy lifestyle. It kick starts your metabolism, regulates appetite, and provides sustained energy for optimal physical and mental performance. By making nutritious choices and including a variety of nutrients, you can harness the power of breakfast to support your weight loss goals and improve your overall health.

The significance of a well-balanced, nutrient-rich Breakfast.

A well-balanced, nutrient-rich breakfast holds immense significance in jumpstarting metabolism and providing sustained energy throughout the day. It serves as the foundation for optimal functioning of the body, supporting weight loss efforts and overall well-being. Metabolism, the process by which the body converts food into energy, tends to be slower in the morning after an overnight fast.

Eating a nutritious breakfast kickstarts metabolism, signaling the body to rev up its energy expenditure. This metabolic boost sets the stage for efficient calorie burning throughout the day, aiding in weight loss and management.

By providing essential nutrients early in the day, breakfast helps stabilize blood sugar levels and prevents energy crashes. A well-balanced breakfast includes a combination of macronutrients such as protein, carbohydrates, and healthy fats. Protein-rich foods like eggs, Greek yogurt, or plant-based alternatives provide amino acids that support muscle maintenance and repair, which in turn boosts metabolism. Complex carbohydrates from whole grains, fruits, and vegetables provide a steady release of energy, sustaining satiety and preventing mid-morning hunger pangs. Healthy fats from sources like nuts, seeds, and avocado contribute to a feeling of fullness and provide sustained energy throughout the day.

In addition to jumpstarting metabolism, breakfast plays a crucial role in providing sustained energy levels. Skipping breakfast or opting for a breakfast lacking in nutrients can lead to energy dips, decreased concentration, and increased cravings for unhealthy foods later in the day. Conversely, a nutrient-rich breakfast supplies the body with the fuel it needs to function optimally. It replenishes glycogen stores in the muscles and liver, ensuring a ready supply of energy for physical and mental activities. This sustained energy prevents overeating later in the day, as individuals are less likely to succumb to cravings and make poor food choices when they are adequately fueled.

Moreover, a well-balanced breakfast sets the tone for healthier eating habits throughout the day. Starting off with a nutrient-rich meal primes the body and mind to make better choices when it comes to subsequent meals and snacks. Research shows that individuals who eat a balanced breakfast are more likely to consume a greater variety of nutrients and make healthier food choices throughout the day. They are less prone to overeating or seeking out high-calorie, sugary foods to compensate for the lack of energy.

Beyond weight loss benefits, a nutritious breakfast supports overall health and well-being. It provides essential vitamins, minerals, and antioxidants necessary for optimal bodily functions. Including fruits, vegetables, and whole grains in breakfast helps meet the recommended daily intake of fiber, promoting healthy digestion, and maintaining a healthy weight. Nutrient-rich breakfasts contribute to stronger immune function, better cognitive performance, improved mood, and enhanced physical endurance.

Furthermore, a well-balanced breakfast positively impacts physical and mental performance. It fuels the brain, improving focus, concentration, and memory. This is especially crucial for students, professionals, or individuals engaging in mentally demanding tasks. Breakfast also enhances physical performance, providing the necessary energy to engage in exercise or daily activities with vigor and stamina.

By jumpstarting metabolism and supplying sustained energy, breakfast can enhance calorie burning and promote weight loss even further when combined with an active lifestyle. In conclusion, a well-balanced, nutrient-rich breakfast plays a vital role in jumpstarting metabolism, providing sustained energy, and supporting overall health and well-being. It sets the stage for optimal bodily functions, promotes weight loss, and enhances physical and mental performance. By prioritizing a nutritious breakfast, individuals can fuel their bodies, regulate appetite, make healthier food choices throughout the day, and embark on a successful weight loss journey while enjoying sustained energy and a heightened sense of well-being.

Purpose Of This Book

The purpose of "Breakfast for a Better Body: Delicious and Nutritious Meal Ideas for Weight Loss" is to empower readers on their weight loss journey by providing them with a diverse range of delicious and healthy breakfast options. This book recognizes that breakfast is a crucial meal for weight loss success and aims to help readers make informed choices about their morning meals. It goes beyond generic suggestions and offers a wide variety of recipes to cater to different tastes and dietary preferences. By presenting a plethora of options, the book ensures that readers can find breakfast ideas that suit their individual needs and preferences, making their weight loss journey more enjoyable and sustainable.

The book's focus on delicious and nutritious breakfast options is designed to debunk the notion that weight loss has to be boring and bland. It encourages readers to view breakfast as an opportunity to indulge in flavorful and satisfying meals while still supporting their weight loss goals. By showcasing recipes that are both tasty and nutrient-rich, the book seeks to create a positive association with breakfast, making it a meal to look forward to rather than a chore.

The recipes featured in the book are carefully crafted to include ingredients that promote weight loss. Each recipe incorporates a balance of macronutrients, such as lean proteins, complex carbohydrates, and healthy fats, to provide sustained energy, support metabolism, and regulate appetite.

By offering a wide array of options, including smoothies, cereal and oatmeal variations, egg-based dishes, and plant-based alternatives, the book caters to different dietary preferences, allowing readers to find breakfast ideas that align with their personal choices.

In addition to recipes, the book provides valuable information and guidance on portion control, mindful eating, and customization options. It encourages readers to explore their creativity and adapt the recipes to suit their taste preferences and dietary needs. The book also emphasizes the importance of incorporating whole grains, fresh fruits, vegetables, and other nutrient-dense ingredients to maximize the nutritional value of breakfast while keeping it satisfying and enjoyable.

By offering a diverse range of breakfast options, the book aims to prevent monotony and boredom often associated with restrictive diets. It promotes the idea that weight loss can be achieved without sacrificing taste and enjoyment.

The recipes presented in the book are not only delicious but also provide the necessary nutrients to fuel the body, support metabolism, and contribute to overall health and well-being.

Ultimately, the purpose of "Breakfast for a Better Body" is to inspire and empower readers to embrace a healthy breakfast routine that supports their weight loss journey. By providing them with a variety of tasty and nutritious breakfast options, the book equips readers with the tools they need to start their day off right, fuel their bodies, and achieve their weight loss goals in a sustainable and enjoyable manner.

Chapter 1: The Breakfast Revolution: Unleashing the Power of a Nutritious Morning Meal

In Chapter 1, "The Breakfast Revolution," we delve into the transformative impact of a nutritious morning meal on our overall health and well-being. This chapter sets the foundation for the book by highlighting the significant role that breakfast plays in our daily lives, specifically in relation to weight loss and wellness.

We begin by exploring the scientific evidence that supports the power of breakfast. We delve into studies that reveal the positive effects of eating a balanced breakfast, such as improved weight management, enhanced metabolism, and increased satiety. We shed light on how breakfast sets the stage for a productive and energized day, boosting physical and mental performance.

To dispel common myths and misconceptions surrounding breakfast and weight loss, we present compelling arguments and evidence. We challenge the notion that skipping breakfast can be a successful weight loss strategy, emphasizing the importance of fueling our bodies with a well-balanced morning meal to support sustainable weight loss efforts.

The chapter includes inspiring success stories from individuals who have experienced the transformative benefits of incorporating a nutritious breakfast into their daily routine. These real-life examples serve as motivation and evidence of the positive impact that a healthy breakfast can have on weight loss and overall well-being.

We delve into the concept of mindful eating and the importance of savoring our breakfast, focusing on the sensory experience of enjoying a nutritious meal. By being present and attentive during breakfast, we can develop a deeper connection with our food, cultivate a healthy relationship with eating, and make mindful choices that align with our weight loss goals.

Throughout the chapter, we emphasize the significance of a well-balanced and nutrient-rich breakfast. We discuss the importance of incorporating macronutrients like protein, carbohydrates, and healthy fats, as well as micronutrients like vitamins, minerals, and antioxidants into our morning meals. By providing our bodies with the essential nutrients it needs, we set ourselves up for success in achieving and maintaining a healthy weight.

In summary, Chapter 1 acts as a comprehensive introduction to the power of breakfast in promoting weight loss and overall well-being. It presents scientific evidence, dispels myths, showcases success stories, and emphasizes the importance of mindful eating.

Scientific research consistently supports the positive impact of breakfast on weight management. Several studies have examined the relationship between breakfast consumption and body weight, providing valuable insights into the benefits of incorporating a nutritious morning meal into our daily routine.

Improved Weight Loss and Weight Maintenance:

Numerous studies have demonstrated that regular breakfast consumption is associated with improved weight loss and weight maintenance. In a randomized controlled trial published in the American Journal of Clinical Nutrition, researchers found that individuals who ate breakfast daily had a greater weight loss and were more successful in long-term weight management compared to those who skipped breakfast.

Increased Metabolic Rate:
Eating breakfast has been shown to increase the metabolic rate, or the number of calories our body burns at rest. Research published in the Journal of the American Dietetic Association reported that individuals who consumed breakfast had a higher resting metabolic rate compared to those who skipped breakfast. This increase in metabolism can aid in calorie burning and support weight loss efforts.

Reduced Caloric Intake:
One of the key benefits of breakfast is its potential to regulate appetite and reduce overall caloric intake throughout the day. Studies have consistently shown that breakfast consumption is associated with lower energy intake and a reduced likelihood of overeating later in the day. In a study published in the International Journal of Obesity, researchers found that individuals who regularly ate breakfast had a lower overall daily energy intake compared to breakfast skippers.

Better Food Choices:
Eating a balanced breakfast has been linked to improved food choices throughout the day. A study published in the Journal of the Academy of Nutrition and Dietetics revealed that individuals who consumed breakfast

had a higher overall diet quality and were more likely to meet the recommended intake of essential nutrients. By starting the day with a nutrient-rich breakfast, individuals are more inclined to make healthier choices and maintain a well-rounded diet.

Impact on Hormones and Blood Sugar Regulation:
Breakfast consumption has been found to influence hormones and blood sugar regulation, which can contribute to weight management. Research published in the journal Obesity Reviews demonstrated that breakfast consumption can lead to improved insulin sensitivity, reduced postprandial glucose response, and better overall glycemic control. These factors play a crucial role in maintaining stable blood sugar levels,

preventing insulin resistance, and supporting weight loss efforts.

Psychological Factors:
Breakfast can have a significant impact on psychological factors related to weight management. Starting the day with a nutritious meal can enhance feelings of satisfaction, reduce cravings, and improve mood. Research published in the International Journal of Endocrinology highlighted the positive effect of breakfast on reducing hunger and increasing satiety, leading to improved control over food intake and decreased likelihood of emotional eating.

Additionally, skipping breakfast or experiencing prolonged fasting can lead to feelings of deprivation and increased vulnerability to unhealthy food choices. A study published in the Journal of Nutritional Science found that individuals who skipped breakfast had a higher preference for high-calorie, sugary foods later in the day, potentially contributing to weight gain.

It Is worth noting that individual differences may exist in the impact of breakfast on weight management. Factors such as age, gender, body composition, and overall dietary habits can influence the outcomes. However, the cumulative evidence consistently points towards the positive role of breakfast in supporting weight loss and weight maintenance.

In conclusion, scientific research provides substantial evidence supporting the positive impact of breakfast on weight management.

Regular breakfast consumption has been associated with improved weight loss, increased metabolic rate, reduced caloric intake, better food choices, regulation of hormones and blood sugar, and positive psychological effects. Incorporating a well-balanced and nutrient-rich breakfast into our daily routine can contribute to a healthier weight and overall well-being.

Debunking Common Myths and Misconceptions Surrounding Breakfast and Weight Loss

Before debunking common myths and misconceptions surrounding breakfast and weight loss, it's essential to acknowledge that there are a variety of beliefs and misconceptions surrounding this topic. Some of these myths can often lead to confusion and misguided practices. Let's explore and debunk a few of the most prevalent myths.

Myth: Skipping breakfast promotes weight loss:

One of the most common misconceptions is that skipping breakfast can aid in weight loss. However, research suggests the opposite. Several studies have shown that individuals who regularly eat a nutritious breakfast are more likely to achieve successful weight loss and weight maintenance. Skipping breakfast can actually lead to increased hunger, overeating later in the day, and potentially making less healthy food choices.

Myth: Eating breakfast leads to overeating throughout the day:
Contrary to popular belief, studies have consistently shown that eating breakfast does not lead to excessive calorie intake later in the day. In fact, individuals who consume a balanced breakfast often have better appetite control, reduced cravings, and a lower likelihood of overeating compared to those who skip breakfast. Starting the day with a nutritious meal can help

regulate hunger and prevent excessive calorie consumption.

Myth: Breakfast must be eaten immediately upon waking up:
While it is ideal to have breakfast within a reasonable timeframe after waking up, there is no specific time constraint that dictates when breakfast should be consumed. The important factor is to prioritize a balanced meal that provides essential nutrients. Some individuals may have time constraints or prefer to delay their first meal of the day, and that is perfectly acceptable as long as they still consume a nutritious breakfast when possible.

Myth: Certain foods can magically boost metabolism:
There is a common belief that specific foods or combinations of foods can

have a significant impact on metabolism and lead to rapid weight loss. While certain foods may have a slight thermogenic effect or temporarily increase metabolic rate, the overall impact on weight loss is minimal. Sustainable weight loss is achieved through a combination of factors, including overall calorie balance, regular physical activity, and adopting a balanced and healthy eating pattern.

Myth: Breakfast is the most important meal of the day for everyone:
While breakfast is indeed an essential meal, its importance can vary depending on individual preferences and lifestyle factors. Some individuals may naturally prefer to skip breakfast or practice intermittent fasting, and as long as their overall nutritional needs

are met throughout the day, it can still lead to successful weight management. It's important to find an eating pattern that works best for an individual's unique needs and preferences.

Myth: Breakfast foods should be low in calories and fat:
There is a misconception that breakfast should consist of low-calorie and low-fat options to promote weight loss. However, incorporating healthy fats into breakfast can be beneficial. Healthy fats, such as those found in avocados, nuts, and seeds, contribute to satiety and help regulate blood sugar levels. Including moderate portions of healthy fats in breakfast can promote feelings of fullness and prevent overeating later in the day.

Myth: Skipping breakfast can "save" calories for later:

Some people believe that skipping breakfast allows them to save calories and eat more throughout the day. However, research suggests that individuals who skip breakfast often compensate by consuming more calories later in the day, particularly in the form of high-sugar and high-fat snacks. This can lead to an overall calorie surplus and hinder weight loss efforts.

Myth: Breakfast should consist of specific "diet" foods:

There is a misconception that breakfast for weight loss should only consist of specific "diet" foods or meal replacements. While incorporating nutrient-dense foods is important, it's equally crucial to focus on variety and enjoyment. A sustainable and balanced breakfast can include whole grains, lean proteins, fruits, vegetables, and dairy or plant-based alternatives. The key is to prioritize real, whole foods that provide essential nutrients and support overall health.

Myth: Breakfast is the only meal that matters for weight loss:
While breakfast is indeed important, weight loss is not solely dependent on this one meal. The overall quality and quantity of calories consumed throughout the day, as well as physical activity levels, play significant roles. It is crucial to maintain a balanced and calorie-controlled diet throughout the entire day, rather than solely relying on breakfast to achieve weight loss goals.

Myth: A small breakfast is sufficient for weight loss:

Some individuals believe that consuming a very small or minimal breakfast is enough for weight loss. However, an excessively small breakfast may not provide the necessary nutrients and energy to sustain the body throughout the day. It is important to strike a balance by consuming a breakfast that is satisfying, nutrient-rich, and appropriately portioned to support weight loss and overall well-being.

Debunking these myths helps to dispel misconceptions and provides a more evidence-based understanding of the role of breakfast in weight loss. A nutritious breakfast can contribute to a healthy eating pattern, support appetite control, and provide sustained energy throughout the day, ultimately aiding in weight management and overall well-being.

Inspiring Success Stories of Individuals who Achieved their Weight loss Goals Through a Healthy Breakfast Routine.

Here are a few inspiring success stories of individuals who achieved their weight loss goals through a healthy breakfast routine:

Sarah's Transformation:
Sarah struggled with weight gain and had difficulty sticking to diets in the past. Determined to make a change, she decided to prioritize a healthy breakfast every morning. She started incorporating a variety of nutrient-rich foods, such as oatmeal topped with

fresh fruits, Greek yogurt, and a sprinkle of nuts. Over time, Sarah noticed increased energy levels and reduced cravings throughout the day. With consistent breakfast habits and a commitment to overall healthier eating, Sarah lost 30 pounds within six months and has successfully maintained her weight loss.

John's Journey:
John had a sedentary lifestyle and struggled with emotional eating. He realized that his breakfast choices were often sugar-laden and lacking in nutrients, leading to energy crashes and poor food choices later in the day. To turn things around, John decided to switch to a balanced breakfast that included a combination of protein, fiber, and healthy fats. He started preparing veggie omelets with

whole-grain toast or overnight oats with chia seeds and berries.

The change in his breakfast routine provided sustained energy, improved his mood, and reduced his cravings. With regular exercise and mindful eating, John lost 50 pounds over the course of a year and experienced a significant improvement in his overall well-being.

Lisa's Balanced Start:
Lisa had struggled with her weight for years and had tried various diets without long-term success. She realized that skipping breakfast and opting for quick, processed snacks throughout the day was hindering her progress.

Determined to make a change, Lisa committed to a nutritious breakfast routine. She began preparing smoothies packed with leafy greens, protein powder, and a variety of fruits. This shift in her breakfast habits set the tone for healthier choices throughout the day. Lisa's energy levels increased, and she found it easier to resist unhealthy temptations.

With a balanced breakfast and an overall lifestyle change, Lisa gradually lost 40 pounds and gained a newfound sense of confidence and well-being.

These success stories demonstrate the transformative power of incorporating a healthy breakfast routine into one's weight loss journey. By prioritizing nutrient-rich foods, managing portion sizes, and establishing sustainable habits, individuals like Sarah, John, and Lisa were able to achieve their weight loss goals and improve their overall health and well-being. These stories serve as inspiration and motivation for others on their own journeys towards a healthier lifestyle. You too can be well on your way to a happier and healthier you by taking inspiration for this stories and using this book as a guide today.

Chapter 2: Designing Your Breakfast Plate: Essential Components for Weight Loss

In Chapter 2, "Designing Your Breakfast Plate: Essential Components for Weight Loss," we delve into the key components that make up a well-balanced breakfast, specifically tailored to support weight loss goals. This chapter focuses on providing readers with practical guidance and actionable steps to create a nutritious and satisfying breakfast that fuels their weight loss journey.

The Power of Protein:
Protein is a crucial component of a weight loss breakfast. It helps to increase feelings of fullness, stabilize blood sugar levels, and preserve lean muscle mass. In this chapter, we

discuss various sources of protein, such as eggs, Greek yogurt, cottage cheese, lean meats, and plant-based options like tofu and legumes. We provide tips on incorporating protein into breakfast recipes and highlight the importance of portion control to ensure a balanced meal.

Fiber for Satiety and Digestive Health: Fiber plays a vital role in weight management by promoting feelings of satiety and supporting healthy digestion. We explore high-fiber options like whole grains, fruits, vegetables, and seeds. By incorporating fiber-rich foods into breakfast, readers can experience prolonged satiety and reduced cravings throughout the day. We also discuss the importance of gradually increasing fiber intake to prevent digestive discomfort.

Healthy Fats for Sustained Energy:
Contrary to popular belief, healthy fats are an essential part of a weight loss breakfast. We explain the benefits of including sources like avocados, nuts, seeds, and olive oil. These healthy fats provide satiety, help regulate blood sugar levels, and contribute to the absorption of fat-soluble vitamins. We guide readers on portion sizes and creative ways to incorporate healthy fats into their breakfast options.

Carbohydrates: Choosing Wisely:
Carbohydrates are an important energy source, but not all carbohydrates are created equal. We discuss the difference between refined carbohydrates and complex carbohydrates, emphasizing the importance of choosing whole grain options like oats, quinoa, and whole

wheat bread. By selecting complex carbohydrates with a low glycemic index, readers can experience sustained energy levels and better blood sugar control.

Nutrient Density: Maximizing Vitamin and Mineral Intake:
A nutrient-dense breakfast is essential for overall health and weight loss. We emphasize the importance of incorporating a variety of colorful fruits and vegetables into breakfast to maximize vitamin and mineral intake.

We highlight specific nutrients that support weight loss efforts, such as vitamin D, calcium, and iron, and provide guidance on selecting breakfast options that are rich in these nutrients.

Portion Control and Mindful Eating:

In this chapter, we also address the significance of portion control and mindful eating during breakfast. We provide practical tips on listening to hunger and fullness cues, avoiding distractions while eating, and savoring each bite.

By practicing portion control and mindful eating, readers can develop a healthier relationship with food, prevent overeating, and support their weight loss goals.

Throughout the chapter, we offer recipe ideas, meal planning tips, and practical strategies for incorporating the essential components discussed. We aim to empower readers to create their own personalized breakfast plates that align with their taste preferences, dietary needs, and weight loss goals.

By understanding the essential components of a weight loss breakfast and learning how to design a well-balanced breakfast plate, readers can set themselves up for success in their weight loss journey. This chapter serves as a comprehensive guide to creating satisfying and nutritious breakfast options that support weight loss, energy levels, and overall well-being.

A well-rounded breakfast that promotes weight loss should include key macronutrients (carbohydrates, protein, and fats) and micronutrients (vitamins and minerals) in appropriate proportions. Let's explore each of these components.

Macronutrients:

a. **Carbohydrates:** Complex carbohydrates provide sustained energy and help keep you feeling full. Opt for whole grain options like oats, quinoa, whole wheat bread, or brown rice. These carbohydrates have a lower glycemic index, which means they have a slower impact on blood sugar levels and provide longer-lasting energy.

b. Protein: Including protein in your breakfast is essential for promoting satiety and preserving muscle mass. Good sources of protein include eggs, Greek yogurt, cottage cheese, lean meats (such as turkey or chicken), legumes (like beans or lentils), and plant-based options like tofu or tempeh.

c. Healthy Fats: Healthy fats are important for their satiating effect and absorption of fat-soluble vitamins. Incorporate sources such as avocados, nuts, seeds, nut butter, and olive oil into your breakfast. However, be mindful of portion sizes, as fats are calorie-dense.

Micronutrients:

a. Vitamins: Breakfast is an excellent opportunity to boost your intake of essential vitamins. Fresh fruits and vegetables are packed with vitamins such as vitamin C, vitamin A, and folate. Include a variety of colorful fruits like berries, citrus fruits, and vegetables like spinach or bell peppers to ensure a wide range of vitamins in your breakfast.

b. Minerals: Micronutrients like iron, calcium, and magnesium are vital for various bodily functions. Iron-rich breakfast options include fortified cereals, spinach, and eggs. Calcium can be obtained from dairy products like milk or yogurt, or plant-based alternatives like fortified plant milks. Magnesium-rich foods include nuts, seeds, and whole grains.

It's important to note that individual nutrient needs may vary based on factors such as age, gender, and activity level. Consulting with a registered dietitian can provide personalized guidance tailored to specific needs and goals.

By incorporating a well-rounded breakfast that includes these key macronutrients and micronutrients, you provide your body with the necessary fuel and nutrients to support weight loss, maintain energy levels, and promote overall health and well-being.

practical tips for portion control and mindful eating.

Portion control and mindful eating are valuable practices that can help promote healthy eating habits and support weight loss goals. Here are some practical tips to incorporate into your breakfast routine.

Use Smaller Plates and Bowls:
Opt for smaller plates and bowls when serving your breakfast. Research suggests that using smaller dishware can help reduce portion sizes and create a visual perception of a fuller plate, which can lead to greater satisfaction with smaller portions.

Measure Ingredients:
To have a better understanding of portion sizes, use measuring cups or a

food scale to measure ingredients, especially for items like cereals, granola, or nut butter. This will help you become more aware of appropriate serving sizes and prevent overconsumption.

Mindful Plating:
Rather than eating directly from containers or packages, take the time to plate your breakfast. This allows you to visualize your portions and be more mindful of what and how much you are eating.

Include a Variety of Foods:
Aim for a well-balanced breakfast that includes a variety of foods from different food groups. By including proteins, whole grains, fruits, and vegetables, you can create a satisfying and nutrient-rich meal. This variety

can help prevent monotony and overeating due to specific food cravings.

Eat Slowly and Chew Thoroughly:
Take the time to enjoy your breakfast and eat slowly. Chew each bite thoroughly before swallowing. Eating at a slower pace allows your brain to register feelings of fullness, which can prevent overeating. It also enhances digestion and nutrient absorption.

Pay Attention to Hunger and Fullness Cues:
Before eating, assess your hunger levels. Are you truly hungry or eating out of habit or emotions? During your meal, pay attention to your body's signals of fullness. Pause periodically to assess your satisfaction and determine

if you need more food or if you are comfortably satisfied.

Minimize Distractions:
Create a calm and focused eating environment by minimizing distractions. Avoid eating in front of screens (such as TVs, computers, or smartphones) as they can lead to mindless eating. Instead, choose a dedicated space for your meals and engage in the sensory experience of eating.

Practice Mindful Snacking:
If you find yourself wanting to snack after breakfast, pause and assess whether you are truly hungry or simply craving something out of habit or boredom. If you genuinely need a snack, opt for nutritious options like fruits, veggies with hummus, or a small

handful of nuts. Be mindful of portion sizes and choose snacks that align with your overall goals.

Keep a Food Journal:
Maintain a food journal or use a mobile app to track your breakfast and overall food intake. This can help increase awareness of your eating patterns, portion sizes, and any emotional or mindless eating habits. It also provides accountability and allows you to reflect on your choices.

Seek Support and Guidance:
Consider working with a registered dietitian or seeking support from a weight loss program or support group. These professionals can provide personalized guidance, help you set realistic goals, and offer strategies to

overcome challenges related to portion control and mindful eating.

Remember, developing healthy eating habits takes time and practice. By incorporating these practical tips into your breakfast routine, you can cultivate a mindful and balanced approach to eating, leading to better portion control, improved satisfaction, and progress towards your weight loss goals.

Customized Breakfast Options for Different Dietary Preferences

When it comes to breakfast, it's important to cater to individual dietary preferences to ensure enjoyment and adherence to a healthy eating plan. Here, we provide guidance on customizing breakfast options for various dietary preferences:

Vegetarian and Vegan Diets:
For those following a vegetarian or vegan diet, there are numerous plant-based options to create a satisfying breakfast. Incorporate protein sources such as tofu, tempeh, legumes (beans, lentils, chickpeas), and plant-based protein powders. Include whole grains like oats, quinoa, or whole wheat bread, as well as a variety of

fruits, vegetables, and nuts for added nutrients and flavors.

Gluten-Free Diets:
For individuals with gluten sensitivities or those following a gluten-free diet, there are many alternatives available. Choose gluten-free grains like rice, quinoa, millet, or certified gluten-free oats. Opt for gluten-free bread, wraps, or cereals. Use alternative flours such as almond flour, coconut flour, or gluten-free flour blends for baking purposes. Ensure all ingredients used are certified gluten-free to avoid cross-contamination.

Paleo or Whole Food Diets:
A paleo or whole food approach emphasizes unprocessed, nutrient-dense foods. Focus on lean protein sources like eggs, poultry, or

fish. Include non-starchy vegetables, fruits, nuts, and seeds. Avoid grains, dairy, and processed sugars. Create breakfast options like vegetable omelets, fruit and nut bowls, or chia seed puddings using natural sweeteners like honey or maple syrup.

Low-Carb or Keto Diets:
For those following a low-carb or ketogenic diet, the emphasis is on reducing carbohydrate intake and increasing healthy fats. Incorporate protein sources like eggs, cottage cheese, or Greek yogurt. Include healthy fats such as avocados, nuts, seeds, coconut oil, or olive oil. Choose low-carb vegetables like leafy greens, broccoli, or cauliflower. Avoid high-carb ingredients like grains, starchy vegetables, and sugars.

Food Allergies and Intolerances:
Individuals with food allergies or intolerances should customize their breakfast options accordingly. Identify and eliminate allergens or trigger foods. Seek alternatives or substitutes for common allergens like dairy, eggs, soy, or nuts. Use dairy-free milk alternatives like almond milk or oat milk. Explore egg replacements like flax or chia eggs. Always check ingredient labels and ensure that your breakfast options are free from allergens.

Specific Dietary Plans:
Certain dietary plans, such as the Mediterranean diet or DASH (Dietary Approaches to Stop Hypertension), have specific guidelines. Customize your breakfast options based on the principles of these plans. Emphasize whole grains, lean proteins, healthy

fats, fruits, and vegetables. Limit sodium and added sugars. Incorporate traditional Mediterranean ingredients like olive oil, olives, or feta cheese.

Here's a detailed guide on customizing your breakfast options based on your dietary preferences.

Vegetarian and Vegan Diets:

Scrambled Tofu: Replace eggs with crumbled tofu seasoned with turmeric, nutritional yeast, and spices. Add vegetables like bell peppers, onions, and spinach for added flavor and nutrients.

Chickpea Flour Pancakes: Use chickpea flour instead of regular flour to make protein-packed pancakes. Top them with fresh fruit or a drizzle of pure maple syrup.

Overnight Chia Pudding: Mix chia seeds with plant-based milk and sweeten with natural sweeteners like agave or stevia. Customize with flavors like cocoa powder, vanilla extract, or fruit puree.

Quinoa Breakfast Bowl: Cook quinoa in plant-based milk and top with nuts, seeds, and berries for a nutrient-dense and protein-rich breakfast.

Veggie Omelet: Prepare an omelet using chickpea flour or tofu as a base and load it with sautéed vegetables, such as mushrooms, zucchini, and spinach.

Vegan Protein Smoothie: Blend plant-based protein powder, frozen fruits, leafy greens, and nut butter with your choice of plant-based milk for a quick and filling breakfast.

Avocado Toast: Spread mashed avocado on whole grain bread and top with sliced tomatoes, sprouts, and a sprinkle of nutritional yeast or sesame seeds.

Vegan Breakfast Burrito: Fill a whole wheat wrap with scrambled tofu, black beans, salsa, and avocado for a satisfying and protein-rich breakfast option.

Vegan Overnight Oats: Combine oats, plant-based milk, chia seeds, and your choice of toppings like fruits, nuts, or coconut flakes. Let it sit overnight for a quick and nutritious breakfast.

Fruit and Nut Butter Wrap: Spread nut butter on a whole wheat tortilla, add sliced fruits like bananas or strawberries, and roll it up for a portable and balanced breakfast.

<u>**Gluten-Free Diets:**</u>

Gluten-Free Oatmeal: Use certified gluten-free oats and prepare oatmeal with your choice of milk. Top with berries, nuts, and a drizzle of honey or pure maple syrup.

Quinoa Breakfast Porridge: Cook quinoa in water or dairy-free milk and add flavors like cinnamon, vanilla extract, and dried fruits for a gluten-free alternative to oatmeal.

Gluten-Free Pancakes: Make pancakes using gluten-free flour blends or alternative flours like almond or coconut flour. Add toppings like fresh fruit or pureed berries.

Yogurt Parfait: Layer dairy-free yogurt with gluten-free granola and fresh fruits for a quick and satisfying breakfast.

Rice Cakes with Nut Butter: Spread nut butter on gluten-free rice cakes and top with sliced fruits or a sprinkle of cinnamon for a crunchy and nutritious breakfast option.

Vegetable Frittata: Use a mixture of eggs or egg substitutes, along with a variety of sautéed vegetables, herbs, and dairy-free cheese for a gluten-free frittata.

Smoothie Bowl: Blend frozen fruits, dairy-free milk, and a protein powder of your choice. Top with gluten-free granola, shredded coconut, and fresh berries for a refreshing and filling breakfast.

Gluten-Free Breakfast Burrito: Wrap scrambled eggs or tofu, avocado, sautéed vegetables, and salsa in a gluten-free tortilla for a satisfying and portable breakfast.

Grain-Free Granola: Make a homemade granola using a combination of nuts, seeds, dried fruits, and sweetened with natural sweeteners like honey or maple syrup.

Gluten-Free Breakfast Muffins: Bake muffins using gluten-free flour blends or almond flour, and customize with additions like fruits, nuts, or dairy-free chocolate chips.

Paleo or Whole Food Diets:

Veggie and Egg Scramble: Sauté a combination of vegetables like peppers, onions, and spinach, and scramble with eggs or egg whites for a nutrient-dense breakfast.

Sweet Potato Hash: Sauté diced sweet potatoes with onions, bell peppers, and your choice of protein like turkey sausage or lean chicken. Serve with a side of fresh fruit.

Paleo Banana Pancakes: Mash ripe bananas and mix them with eggs, almond flour, and a dash of cinnamon. Cook as pancakes and serve with almond butter and fresh berries.

Coconut Milk Chia Pudding: Mix chia seeds with coconut milk and a natural sweetener like honey or maple syrup. Let it sit overnight and top with sliced almonds and coconut flakes.

Green Smoothie: Blend a combination of leafy greens, coconut milk or water, a scoop of protein powder, and a handful of frozen fruits for a nutritious and paleo-friendly breakfast.

Salmon and Avocado Roll-Ups: Spread mashed avocado on smoked salmon slices and roll them up for a protein-rich and satisfying breakfast.

Almond Flour Muffins: Bake muffins using almond flour and sweeten with honey or mashed bananas. Customize with additions like blueberries, chopped nuts, or shredded coconut.

Vegetable Omelet with Coconut Oil: Cook an omelet using coconut oil and fill it with a variety of sautéed vegetables like mushrooms, spinach, and tomatoes.

Paleo Breakfast Bowl: Combine roasted sweet potatoes, scrambled eggs, avocado slices, and nitrate-free bacon for a hearty and nutritious breakfast.

Mixed Berry Salad with Nuts: Toss together a mix of fresh berries, such as strawberries, blueberries, and raspberries, with a handful of nuts for a refreshing and nutrient-dense breakfast option.

<u>Low-Carb or Keto Diets:</u>

Egg and Vegetable Muffins: Beat eggs with a variety of chopped vegetables like bell peppers, spinach, and mushrooms. Pour the mixture into muffin tins and bake for a protein-packed breakfast option.

Greek Yogurt with Nuts and Seeds: Enjoy full-fat Greek yogurt topped with a handful of mixed nuts and seeds for a low-carb and high-protein breakfast.

Smoked Salmon Roll-Ups: Spread cream cheese on smoked salmon slices and roll them up with cucumber or avocado slices for a delicious and keto-friendly breakfast.

Coconut Flour Pancakes: Use coconut flour instead of regular flour to make fluffy pancakes. Serve with sugar-free syrup and a pat of butter for a low-carb option.

Green Vegetable Smoothie: Blend a combination of leafy greens, avocado, cucumber, and coconut milk for a refreshing and low-carb breakfast option.

Bacon and Egg Breakfast Skillet: Cook bacon and eggs in a skillet with sautéed vegetables like onions and bell peppers for a hearty and keto-friendly breakfast.

Avocado and Egg Boats: Cut an avocado in half, remove the pit, and crack an egg into each half. Bake until the egg is cooked to your liking and top with salt, pepper, and any desired herbs or spices.

Cauliflower Hash Browns: Grate cauliflower and sauté it in olive oil until lightly browned. Season with salt, pepper, and your choice of herbs and spices for a low-carb alternative to traditional hash browns.

Keto Chia Seed Pudding: Mix chia seeds with unsweetened almond milk, a sugar substitute like stevia or erythritol, and flavorings like vanilla extract or cocoa powder. Let it sit in the refrigerator overnight for a satisfying and low-carb breakfast.

Spinach and Feta Egg Muffins: Whisk together eggs, chopped spinach, crumbled feta cheese, and seasonings. Pour the mixture into muffin tins and bake until set for a portable and protein-rich breakfast option.

Almond Flour Breakfast Biscuits: Use almond flour as the base for homemade biscuits and enjoy them with butter, sugar-free jam, or your preferred low-carb spreads.

Keto Breakfast Burrito: Wrap scrambled eggs, cooked bacon or sausage, cheese, and avocado in a large lettuce leaf or low-carb tortilla for a protein-packed and low-carb breakfast.

Zucchini Noodle Breakfast Bowl: Spiralize zucchini into noodles and sauté them with garlic and olive oil. Top with a poached egg and grated Parmesan cheese for a light and flavorful low-carb breakfast.

Low-Carb Smoothie: Blend unsweetened almond milk or coconut milk, a handful of low-carb fruits like berries or avocado, a scoop of low-carb protein powder, and a natural sugar substitute if desired.

Keto Veggie Scramble: Sauté a mix of low-carb vegetables like zucchini, bell peppers, and mushrooms in olive oil. Add beaten eggs and cook until set, creating a delicious and filling breakfast dish.

Food Allergies and Intolerances:

When dealing with food allergies and intolerances, it's essential to customize breakfast options to suit your specific needs. Here are some suggestions for catering to food allergies and intolerances.

Dairy-Free Options:

Swap dairy milk with plant-based alternatives like almond milk, coconut milk, or oat milk in your cereal, smoothies, or coffee.

Use dairy-free yogurt made from soy, coconut, or almond milk as a base for parfaits or smoothie bowls.

Substitute butter with dairy-free alternatives like coconut oil, avocado, or olive oil for cooking and spreading on toast.

Egg-Free Options:

Create an egg-free omelet by using chickpea flour or tofu as a base and adding sautéed vegetables, herbs, and spices.

Use egg replacers like mashed banana, applesauce, or flaxseed meal mixed

with water in baking recipes for pancakes, muffins, or bread.
Explore plant-based protein options like lentils, chickpeas, or tempeh to provide a protein-rich component to your breakfast.

Soy-Free Options:
Substitute soy milk or tofu with other plant-based alternatives like almond milk, oat milk, or hemp milk in recipes or beverages.
Use alternative protein sources like quinoa, chia seeds, hemp seeds, or pea protein powder to ensure a balanced and complete breakfast.

Nut-Free Options:
Replace nut butters with seed butters such as sunflower seed butter or pumpkin seed butter on toast, rice cakes, or in smoothies.

Incorporate seeds like chia seeds, hemp seeds, or flaxseeds into your breakfast options for added nutrition and texture. Choose cereals or granola that are free from nuts or processed in a nut-free facility to avoid cross-contamination.

Gluten-Free Options:
Opt for gluten-free grains like quinoa, rice, buckwheat, or certified gluten-free oats as the base for your breakfast bowls or porridge.
Use gluten-free flour blends or alternative flours like almond flour, coconut flour, or tapioca flour in baking recipes for pancakes, waffles, or muffins.

Check labels to ensure that packaged foods like cereals, granola, or bread are certified gluten-free and free from gluten-containing ingredients.

Specific Allergens:
Read food labels carefully to identify potential allergens and avoid them in your breakfast choices. Prepare homemade breakfast options using fresh, whole ingredients to have full control over the ingredients and allergens present.

Remember to adjust portion sizes and ingredient quantities to align with your specific dietary needs and goals. It's always a good idea to consult with a registered dietitian or healthcare professional to ensure that your customized breakfast options are appropriate for your individual requirements.

Chapter 3: Rise and Shine with Energy-Boosting Smoothies

In this chapter, we delve into the world of energy-boosting smoothies, offering a refreshing and nutritious way to start your day. Smoothies are a fantastic breakfast option as they allow for a quick and convenient meal while packing a punch of essential nutrients. We explore a variety of smoothie recipes that will invigorate your mornings and keep you fueled throughout the day.

Smoothies provide an excellent opportunity to incorporate an abundance of fruits and vegetables into your diet, delivering a wide range of vitamins, minerals, and antioxidants. Whether you prefer fruit-based or green smoothies, we have a selection of recipes to suit your taste buds and nutritional needs.

We focus on low-sugar options, utilizing the natural sweetness of fruits or adding minimal amounts of natural sweeteners like honey or maple syrup. By avoiding excessive added sugars, our smoothies provide sustained energy without causing spikes in blood sugar levels.

To enhance the nutritional profile of our smoothies, we explore the addition of protein sources, such as Greek yogurt, plant-based protein powders, or nut butters. Protein helps to promote satiety, support muscle recovery, and stabilize blood sugar levels, making it an essential component of a well-rounded breakfast.

Incorporating healthy fats into smoothies is another way to boost their nutritional value. We introduce options like avocado, coconut milk, or chia seeds, which provide omega-3 fatty acids and contribute to a creamy texture. Healthy fats aid in nutrient absorption and help you feel satisfied for longer, promoting portion control and preventing overeating later in the day.

Additionally, we discuss the benefits of incorporating superfoods into your smoothies. Superfoods like spinach, kale, berries, or spirulina are rich in antioxidants and phytochemicals, which support overall health and contribute to a strong immune system. These additions can elevate the nutritional value of your smoothies and provide an extra health boost.

Throughout this chapter, we provide easy-to-follow recipes and offer suggestions for ingredient substitutions and variations to suit different taste preferences and dietary restrictions. With our energy-boosting smoothies, you can enjoy a delicious and nutrient-dense breakfast that fuels your body, supports weight loss, and kickstarts your day on a healthy note.

Introducing Variety of nutrient-packed smoothie recipes

We introduce a variety of smoothie recipes that are not only delicious but also packed with essential nutrients, making them the perfect choice for a healthy and satisfying breakfast. These recipes have been carefully curated to provide a balance of carbohydrates, protein, healthy fats, vitamins, and minerals to help you kickstart your day on a nutritious note.

Tropical Green Delight: This refreshing smoothie combines the goodness of leafy greens like spinach or kale with tropical fruits like pineapple, mango, and coconut water. It's loaded with antioxidants, fiber, and vitamin C, providing a burst of energy to start your day.

Berry Blast: Bursting with vibrant colors and flavors, this smoothie incorporates a mix of antioxidant-rich berries such as blueberries, strawberries, and raspberries. Add in a scoop of Greek yogurt or a plant-based protein powder to boost the protein content and make it more filling.

Banana Almond Power: This smoothie combines the creaminess of bananas with the richness of almond butter and almond milk. It's a great source of potassium, healthy fats, and protein, keeping you satisfied and energized throughout the morning.

Chocolate Banana Protein: For all the chocolate lovers out there, this smoothie is a treat! It combines ripe bananas, a scoop of chocolate protein powder, almond milk, and a spoonful of cacao powder for a nutritious and indulgent breakfast option. It provides a good dose of protein and satisfies your sweet cravings.

Green Protein Boost: Packed with nutrient-dense ingredients, this smoothie features a mix of leafy greens, like spinach or kale, along with a plant-based protein powder, a tablespoon of chia seeds, and a handful of mixed berries. It's a perfect way to fuel your body with plant-based protein, fiber, and antioxidants.

Peanut Butter Banana Bliss: This classic combination of peanut butter and bananas creates a smoothie that is both creamy and delicious. Add a dash of cinnamon and a tablespoon of flaxseed for added fiber and omega-3 fatty acids. It's a great option for a quick and satisfying breakfast.

Mango Coconut Dream: Transport yourself to a tropical paradise with this smoothie that combines ripe mango, coconut milk, a scoop of vanilla protein powder, and a handful of spinach. It's a delightful blend of flavors and provides a good amount of fiber, vitamins, and minerals.

Matcha Green Tea Boost: For a morning pick-me-up, try this smoothie featuring matcha green tea powder, almond milk, a frozen banana, and a teaspoon of honey or maple syrup for sweetness. Matcha is known for its high concentration of antioxidants and provides a gentle energy boost without the crash.

Pina Colada Paradise: Indulge in the tropical flavors of pineapple, coconut milk, and a splash of lime juice. You can also add a scoop of vanilla protein powder for an extra protein punch. This smoothie is a refreshing way to start your day and reminds you of a beach getaway.

Chai Spice Smoothie: This smoothie combines the warmth and richness of chai spices like cinnamon, ginger, and nutmeg with a blend of almond milk, banana, and a scoop of vanilla protein powder. It's a flavorful and aromatic way to fuel your morning.

Avocado Blueberry Blast: Creamy avocado, antioxidant-rich blueberries, and a splash of almond milk come together in this smoothie. It's a powerhouse of healthy fats, vitamins, and fiber, providing a satisfying and nourishing breakfast option.

Mocha Protein Shake: If you love the combination of coffee and chocolate, this smoothie is for you. Blend a shot of espresso or strong coffee with a scoop of chocolate protein powder, almond milk, and a tablespoon of unsweetened cocoa powder. It's a great way to get a boost of caffeine and protein in the morning.

Green Detox Smoothie: This smoothie is a refreshing blend of cucumber, kale or spinach, green apple, lemon juice, and coconut water. It's a hydrating and detoxifying option that helps to alkalize the body and provide a wealth of vitamins and minerals.

Raspberry Beet Power Smoothie: Beets are known for their natural sweetness and vibrant color. Combine them with raspberries, a handful of spinach, a tablespoon of flaxseeds, and almond milk for a nutrient-packed smoothie. It's high in antioxidants, fiber, and essential nutrients.

These diverse smoothie recipes offer a range of flavors and ingredients to suit different taste preferences. They can be customized by adjusting the sweetness, thickness, or adding additional superfoods like hemp seeds, spirulina, or goji berries. Whether you're looking for a fruity blend, a protein-packed option, or a detoxifying choice, these smoothies will provide you with a nourishing and energizing start to your day.

Low-sugar and high-fiber options

Here we provide options for both fruit-based and green smoothies, ensuring a diverse range of choices to suit different preferences. Our focus is on using low-sugar and high-fiber ingredients to maximize the nutritional benefits of these smoothies.

Fruit-based smoothies are a delicious and refreshing way to incorporate a variety of fruits into your breakfast routine. We recommend using whole fruits, such as berries, citrus fruits, apples, and bananas, as they provide natural sweetness and fiber. By using whole fruits instead of fruit juices or processed sweeteners, we can minimize added sugars and increase the fiber content of the smoothies.

To enhance the fiber content even further, we suggest adding sources of soluble fiber, such as chia seeds, flaxseeds, or oats, to your fruit-based smoothies. These ingredients not only contribute to a thicker and more filling texture but also help regulate blood sugar levels and support healthy digestion.

Green smoothies, on the other hand, are an excellent way to boost your intake of leafy greens and other vegetables. We recommend using a base of leafy greens like spinach, kale, or Swiss chard, as they are rich in fiber, vitamins, and minerals. Combining these greens with fruits like pineapple, mango, or green apple adds sweetness and masks any potential bitterness.

To keep the sugar content low in green smoothies, we advise limiting the amount of fruit used and focusing on incorporating more non-starchy vegetables. This approach ensures that you're still getting the natural sweetness from fruits while maintaining a balanced and nutrient-dense smoothie.

Additionally, we suggest including high-fiber ingredients like hemp seeds, avocado, or psyllium husk in your green smoothies. These ingredients not only contribute to a creamy texture but also provide additional fiber, healthy fats, and essential nutrients.

Here are some smoothie recipes, fruit-based and green smoothies, that focus on low-sugar and high-fiber ingredients:

Mixed Berry Bliss (Fruit-Based Smoothie):

1 cup mixed berries (such as strawberries, blueberries, and raspberries)

1/2 ripe banana

1 cup spinach or kale

1 tablespoon chia seeds

1 cup unsweetened almond milk

Instructions: Blend all the ingredients until smooth and creamy. Adjust the consistency by adding more almond milk if desired.

Green Goddess (Green Smoothie):

1 cup spinach

1/2 ripe avocado

1/2 cucumber, peeled

1/2 green apple

1 tablespoon fresh lemon juice

1 tablespoon ground flaxseeds

1 cup coconut water or unsweetened almond milk

Instructions: Blend all the ingredients until well combined and creamy. Add more liquid if needed to achieve your desired consistency.

Detox Green Dream (Green Smoothie):
1 cup kale or spinach
1 small green apple, cored and chopped
1/2 cucumber, peeled
1/2 lemon, juiced
1/2-inch piece of ginger, grated
1 tablespoon hemp seeds
1 cup coconut water or unsweetened almond milk

Instructions: Blend all the ingredients until smooth and creamy. Adjust the consistency by adding more liquid if desired.

Green Mango Tango:

1 cup spinach

1 cup chopped ripe mango

1/2 ripe banana

1 tablespoon ground flaxseeds

1 cup unsweetened coconut water or almond milk

Instructions: Blend all the ingredients until smooth and creamy. Adjust the consistency by adding more liquid if desired.

Berry Avocado Blast:

1 cup mixed berries (such as strawberries, blueberries, and blackberries)

1/4 ripe avocado

1 tablespoon chia seeds

1 tablespoon almond butter

1 cup unsweetened almond milk

Instructions: Blend all the ingredients until well combined and creamy. Add more liquid if needed to reach your desired consistency.

Chocolate Peanut Butter Powerhouse:
1 cup spinach or kale
1 tablespoon unsweetened cocoa powder
1 tablespoon natural peanut butter
1 tablespoon ground flaxseeds
1 cup unsweetened almond milk
1/2 frozen banana
Instructions: Blend all the ingredients until smooth and creamy. Adjust the consistency by adding more almond milk if desired.

Incorporating these low-sugar and high-fiber smoothies into your breakfast routine will not only provide a tasty and refreshing start to your day but also help support your weight loss goals and overall health. Enjoy the benefits of these nutrient-packed beverages and get creative by trying different combinations to find your favorite smoothie recipes.

Adding protein, healthy fats, and superfoods

Smoothies are incredibly versatile, allowing you to customize them to suit your taste preferences and nutritional needs. Here are some suggestions for adding protein, healthy fats, and superfoods to your smoothies.

Protein Boost:

Add a scoop of protein powder: Choose from options like whey protein, plant-based protein (such as pea, hemp, or rice protein), or collagen peptides. Protein powder helps to increase satiety, support muscle recovery, and promote weight loss.

Greek yogurt or cottage cheese: These dairy-based options provide a creamy texture and a good source of protein.

Silken tofu: Blend in a few cubes of silken tofu to add a protein punch without altering the taste.

Nut butter: Add a tablespoon of almond butter, peanut butter, or cashew butter for a delicious protein and flavor boost.

<u>**Healthy Fat Additions:**</u>

Avocado: Incorporate half a ripe avocado for a creamy texture and a dose of heart-healthy monounsaturated fats.

Chia seeds: These tiny powerhouses are rich in omega-3 fatty acids and fiber, which helps to promote fullness and support digestion.

Flaxseeds: Grind flaxseeds and sprinkle them into your smoothie for added omega-3s and fiber.

Coconut oil or coconut milk: These provide healthy fats and a touch of tropical flavor.

Nuts or seeds: Add a handful of almonds, walnuts, pumpkin seeds, or sunflower seeds for a satisfying crunch and extra nutrients.

Superfood Boosters:

Spinach or kale: Sneak in a handful of leafy greens for a boost of vitamins, minerals, and antioxidants.

Spirulina or chlorella powder: These nutrient-dense algae powders are rich in protein, vitamins, and minerals.

Matcha powder: Add a teaspoon of matcha powder for an antioxidant boost and a natural source of caffeine.

Acai berry or maqui berry powder: These antioxidant-rich powders can add a vibrant purple hue and a burst of flavor to your smoothie.

Cacao nibs or powder: Sprinkle in some cacao nibs or use unsweetened cocoa powder for a rich chocolatey taste and a dose of antioxidants.

Remember to adjust the quantities based on your preferences and consult any specific dietary guidelines or restrictions you may have. Adding protein, healthy fats, and superfoods to your smoothies not only enhances their nutritional value but also contributes to a more balanced and satisfying meal.

By incorporating these suggestions, you can transform your smoothies into nutrient-packed powerhouses that support your weight loss journey and provide a wide range of health benefits. Experiment with different combinations to find your favorite additions and enjoy the versatility and nourishment that smoothies have to offer.

Chapter 4: From the Grains to Glory: Wholesome Cereal and Oatmeal Delights

In this chapter, we delve into the world of wholesome cereal and oatmeal breakfast options that will delight your taste buds and support your weight loss goals. These recipes are designed to provide a balanced combination of complex carbohydrates, fiber, protein, and healthy fats to keep you satiated and energized throughout the morning.

Creative Cereal Combinations:
We explore creative and nutritious cereal combinations that go beyond the typical store-bought options. From homemade granola made with whole grains, nuts, and seeds to a variety of mixed cereals, you'll discover how to create your own delicious cereal blends

while avoiding added sugars and artificial ingredients.

Nourishing Oatmeal Creations:
Oatmeal is a breakfast classic that can be transformed into a nutritious and satisfying meal. We share a range of oatmeal recipes, including overnight oats, stove-top oatmeal, and baked oatmeal. These recipes incorporate different flavors and toppings, such as fresh fruits, nuts, seeds, and spices, to keep your breakfasts interesting and flavorful.

Exploring Alternative Grains:
We introduce you to the world of alternative grains like quinoa, amaranth, and millet. These grains offer a variety of textures and flavors while providing a rich source of nutrients. You'll learn how to

incorporate these grains into your breakfast routine to add diversity and maximize the nutritional value of your meals.

Sweeteners and Toppings:
We discuss the importance of choosing natural sweeteners like honey, maple syrup, or dates instead of refined sugars. We also explore healthier alternatives like stevia or monk fruit sweeteners for those who prefer a low-calorie option. Additionally, we provide a range of nutritious toppings such as fresh fruits, yogurt, nuts, and seeds to add texture, flavor, and additional nutrients to your cereal and oatmeal bowls.

Preparing Ahead and On-the-Go Options:

We understand the need for convenience in our busy lives. In this chapter, we provide tips and techniques for prepping your cereal and oatmeal ahead of time, making it easier to enjoy a nutritious breakfast even on hectic mornings. We also share on-the-go options like portable oatmeal cups, cereal bars, and smoothie bowls that you can take with you when time is limited.

By exploring the world of wholesome cereals and oatmeal delights, you'll have a wide range of delicious options to choose from that support your weight loss journey. These recipes will provide you with the necessary nutrients to fuel your body, keep you satisfied, and help you maintain a healthy and balanced lifestyle. Get ready to enjoy the comforting and nourishing benefits of these grain-based breakfast creations!

Creative and nutritious cereal and oatmeal recipes

Creative and nutritious cereal and oatmeal recipes offer a delicious and satisfying way to start your day while providing essential nutrients. These recipes go beyond traditional options and incorporate wholesome ingredients to support your weight loss journey.
Here are some creative and nutritious cereal and oatmeal recipes.

Homemade Nutty Granola:
Ingredients:
2 cups rolled oats

1 cup mixed nuts (almonds, walnuts, pecans), chopped
1/4 cup pumpkin seeds
1/4 cup sunflower seeds
2 tablespoons chia seeds
2 tablespoons flaxseeds
1/4 cup pure maple syrup
2 tablespoons coconut oil, melted
1 teaspoon vanilla extract
1/2 teaspoon cinnamon
Pinch of salt
Instructions:

Preheat the oven to 325°F (165°C) and line a baking sheet with parchment paper.

In a large mixing bowl, combine the oats, nuts, seeds, cinnamon, and salt.

In a separate bowl, whisk together the maple syrup, melted coconut oil, and vanilla extract.

Pour the wet mixture over the dry ingredients and mix well until everything is evenly coated.

Spread the granola mixture onto the prepared baking sheet in an even layer.

Bake for 20-25 minutes, stirring occasionally, until the granola turns golden brown and crispy.

Remove from the oven and let it cool completely before storing in an airtight container.

Apple Cinnamon Overnight Oats:
Ingredients:

1/2 cup rolled oats
1/2 cup unsweetened almond milk (or any milk of your choice)
1/4 cup unsweetened applesauce
1 tablespoon chia seeds
1 tablespoon pure maple syrup
1/2 teaspoon cinnamon
1/4 teaspoon vanilla extract
1 small apple, diced
Optional toppings: chopped nuts, raisins, cinnamon

Instructions:

In a jar or container, combine the oats, almond milk, applesauce, chia seeds, maple syrup, cinnamon, and vanilla extract.

Stir well to mix all the ingredients together.

Add the diced apple and gently mix it into the oat mixture.

Cover the jar/container and refrigerate overnight or for at least 4 hours.

In the morning, give the oats a good stir and add your desired toppings.

Enjoy the apple cinnamon overnight oats cold or heat them in the microwave for a warm breakfast.

<u>Quinoa Breakfast Bowl:</u>
Ingredients:

1/2 cup cooked quinoa
1/4 cup Greek yogurt
1/4 cup mixed berries (strawberries, blueberries, raspberries)
1 tablespoon honey or pure maple syrup
1 tablespoon sliced almonds

1 tablespoon unsweetened shredded coconut

Optional toppings: chia seeds, hemp seeds, pumpkin seeds

Instructions:

In a bowl, layer the cooked quinoa and Greek yogurt.

Top with mixed berries, drizzle with honey or maple syrup.

Sprinkle with sliced almonds and shredded coconut.

Add any additional toppings of your choice.

Mix everything together just before eating to combine the flavors and textures.

Crunchy Nutty Granola:

2 cups rolled oats

1/2 cup chopped nuts (such as almonds, walnuts, or pecans)

1/4 cup seeds (such as pumpkin seeds or sunflower seeds)

2 tablespoons honey or maple syrup

1 tablespoon coconut oil, melted

1 teaspoon vanilla extract

Pinch of salt

Instructions: Preheat the oven to 325°F (165°C). In a bowl, combine oats, nuts, seeds, honey or maple syrup, melted coconut oil, vanilla extract, and salt. Mix until everything is well coated. Spread the mixture on a lined baking sheet and bake for 20-25 minutes, stirring occasionally, until golden brown. Allow it to cool completely before storing in an airtight container.

Berry Parfait:

1/2 cup Greek yogurt

1/4 cup granola (store-bought or homemade)

1/4 cup mixed berries (such as strawberries, blueberries, and raspberries)

1 tablespoon honey or maple syrup

Instructions: In a glass or bowl, layer Greek yogurt, granola, and mixed berries. Drizzle with honey or maple syrup. Repeat the layers if desired. Serve immediately and enjoy!

Chocolate Peanut Butter Overnight Oats:

1/2 cup rolled oats

1/2 cup almond milk (or any milk of choice)

1 tablespoon cocoa powder

1 tablespoon peanut butter

1 tablespoon honey or maple syrup

Optional toppings: sliced banana, chopped nuts, or chocolate chips

Instructions: In a jar or container, combine oats, almond milk, cocoa powder, peanut butter, and sweetener. Mix well. Cover and refrigerate overnight. In the morning, give it a good stir, and add your desired toppings. Enjoy cold or heat it up in the microwave if desired.

Savory Quinoa Breakfast Bowl:
1/2 cup cooked quinoa
1/4 cup sautéed vegetables (such as bell peppers, spinach, or mushrooms)
1/4 cup cooked black beans
1 fried or poached egg
Optional toppings: sliced avocado, salsa, or a sprinkle of cheese
Instructions: In a bowl, combine cooked quinoa, sautéed vegetables, and black beans. Top with a fried or poached egg and your desired toppings. Season with salt, pepper, and any other preferred spices. Enjoy warm.

Coconut Chia Pudding:

1/4 cup chia seeds

1 cup coconut milk (canned or homemade)

1 tablespoon honey or maple syrup

1/4 teaspoon vanilla extract

Optional toppings: fresh berries, shredded coconut, or crushed nuts

Instructions: In a bowl, mix chia seeds, coconut milk, honey or maple syrup, and vanilla extract. Stir well to combine. Let it sit for 10 minutes, then stir again to prevent clumping. Cover and refrigerate for at least 2 hours or overnight until it thickens. Serve chilled with your preferred toppings.

Yogurt Parfait:

1/2 cup Greek yogurt

1/4 cup granola

1/4 cup mixed fresh fruits (such as sliced strawberries, diced mango, or kiwi)

Optional toppings: drizzle of honey or maple syrup, a sprinkle of cinnamon or nutmeg

Instructions: In a glass or bowl, layer Greek yogurt, granola, and mixed fresh fruits. Repeat the layers if desired. Top with your preferred toppings. Serve immediately and enjoy!

With these creative and satisfying cereal and oatmeal recipes, you can start your day on a delicious and nutritious note. Enjoy the variety of flavors, textures, and customizable options as you explore the world of breakfast cereals and oatmeal.

Incorporate a range of grains to add diversity and maximize nutritional value.

Incorporating a range of grains like quinoa, amaranth, and millet into your breakfast options can add diversity to your meals and maximize their nutritional value. These grains offer unique flavors, textures, and health benefits that can enhance your overall breakfast experience.

Quinoa:

Quinoa is a complete protein and is rich in fiber, vitamins, and minerals. It provides a hearty and satisfying base for breakfast bowls or can be cooked into a creamy porridge. Try incorporating cooked quinoa into your oatmeal, adding it to smoothies, or using it as a topping for yogurt to boost the protein content and add a nutty flavor.

Amaranth:

Amaranth is another nutritious grain that is gluten-free and rich in fiber, protein, and micronutrients. It has a slightly sweet and earthy taste and can be cooked into a creamy porridge or added to granola mixes for extra crunch. Consider combining amaranth with other grains or using it as a substitute for oats in recipes to add variety to your breakfast routine.

Millet:

Millet is a versatile grain that is gluten-free and provides a good source of protein, fiber, and essential minerals like magnesium and phosphorus. It has a mild, nutty flavor and can be cooked into a fluffy and creamy consistency, similar to rice. Millet can be used in porridges, breakfast bakes, or as a base for grain-based breakfast bowls, adding a delightful texture and nutty taste.

Buckwheat:
Despite its name, buckwheat is not related to wheat and is naturally gluten-free. It is a good source of fiber, protein, and essential minerals. Use buckwheat flour to make pancakes or waffles, or cook buckwheat groats as a hearty breakfast porridge.

Teff:
Teff is a tiny grain that is native to Ethiopia and is gluten-free. It is high in fiber, iron, and calcium. Use teff flour to make delicious pancakes or

incorporate cooked teff grains into porridge or breakfast bowls.

When incorporating these diverse grains into your breakfast, ensure that you choose whole grain options rather than refined grains. Whole grains retain the bran, germ, and endosperm, making them higher in fiber and nutrients. Additionally, be mindful of added sugars in your breakfast choices. Opt for natural sweeteners like fruits, spices, or a small drizzle of honey or maple syrup, if desired, instead of processed sugars.

Choose whole grains and avoiding added sugars in packaged cereals for optimal nutrition

Choosing whole grains and avoiding added sugars in packaged cereals is crucial for optimizing your breakfast's nutritional value and supporting your overall health. Here are detailed explanations on the importance of these choices.

Whole Grains:

a) Fiber Powerhouse: Whole grains are rich in dietary fiber, which offers numerous health benefits. Fiber aids in digestion, promotes a feeling of fullness, and helps regulate blood sugar levels. It also supports a healthy gut microbiome and can contribute to weight management.

b) Essential Nutrients: Whole grains provide a wide range of essential nutrients, including B vitamins, vitamin E, magnesium, selenium, and zinc. These nutrients play crucial roles in energy production, immune function, and cell maintenance.

c) Heart Health: Consuming whole grains has been associated with a reduced risk of heart disease. The fiber, antioxidants, and phytochemicals found in whole grains help lower cholesterol levels, maintain healthy blood pressure, and support cardiovascular health.

Added Sugars in Packaged Cereals:

a) Empty Calories: Many packaged cereals are loaded with added sugars, which provide little to no nutritional value. Consuming excessive amounts of added sugars can contribute to weight gain, increase the risk of chronic diseases, and negatively impact overall health.

b) Blood Sugar Control: Foods high in added sugars can cause a rapid spike in blood sugar levels, leading to energy crashes and increased cravings. This can make it challenging to maintain stable energy levels and can contribute to the development of insulin resistance and type 2 diabetes.

c) Nutrient Dilution: Cereals high in added sugars often lack essential nutrients found in whole grains. By consuming these sugary cereals, you miss out on the beneficial fiber, vitamins, and minerals that whole grains provide.

When selecting packaged cereals, it's essential to read labels carefully and make informed choices:

a) **Look for Whole Grain Options:** Choose cereals that list whole grains as the first ingredient, such as whole wheat, whole oats, or whole barley. Avoid cereals that list refined grains, such as enriched flour or sugar, as the primary ingredients.

b) **Watch out for Added Sugars:** Check the nutrition label for added sugars. Be cautious of cereals that have high sugar content or multiple forms of added sugars, such as corn syrup, honey, or molasses.

c) **Portion Control:** Even if a cereal is made with whole grains and has limited added sugars, be mindful of portion sizes to avoid excessive calorie intake. Stick to recommended serving sizes and consider adding nutrient-rich toppings, like fresh fruit or nuts, for added flavor and nutritional value.

By choosing whole grain cereals and avoiding those with added sugars, you can enjoy a nutritious breakfast that supports weight management, provides essential nutrients, and promotes overall health.

Chapter 5: Egg-Cellent Creations: Protein-Packed Breakfasts

In this chapter, we delve into the world of protein-packed breakfasts featuring eggs. Eggs are a versatile and nutrient-dense food that can be enjoyed in various delicious ways. Here, we will highlight the benefits of incorporating eggs into your breakfast routine and provide ideas for creating protein-rich meals.

High-Quality Protein: Eggs are known for their high-quality protein content. They contain all essential amino acids, making them a complete protein source. Protein is essential for building and repairing tissues, supporting muscle growth, and maintaining satiety, which can be especially beneficial for weight loss.

Satiety and Weight Management: Including protein-rich foods like eggs in your breakfast can help keep you feeling full and satisfied throughout the morning. This can prevent overeating later in the day and support weight management efforts. Eggs have been shown to enhance feelings of satiety and reduce calorie intake in subsequent meals.

Nutrient Profile: Eggs are a nutrient powerhouse. They are rich in vitamins such as vitamin B12, vitamin D, vitamin A, and folate. They also provide minerals like iron, zinc, and selenium, which are important for various bodily functions. Additionally, eggs contain beneficial antioxidants like lutein and zeaxanthin, which promote eye health.

Versatility in Cooking: Eggs can be prepared in numerous ways, allowing for a variety of protein-packed breakfast options. Whether you prefer scrambled eggs, omelets, frittatas, or egg muffins, there are endless possibilities to cater to your taste preferences and dietary needs.

Vegetarian Options: Eggs can be a valuable protein source for vegetarians. They offer an alternative to meat-based proteins and can be incorporated into vegetarian breakfast options like vegetable-filled omelets or egg-based breakfast wraps.

Nutrient Pairing: Combining eggs with other nutrient-rich ingredients can further enhance the nutritional value of your breakfast. You can add vegetables, herbs, and spices to boost flavor and increase the vitamin and mineral content. Pairing eggs with whole grain toast or incorporating them into a breakfast salad adds additional fiber and complex carbohydrates to create a balanced meal.

Customization: One of the great aspects of egg-based breakfasts is their versatility. You can personalize your meal by adding a variety of ingredients such as spinach, tomatoes, mushrooms, bell peppers, cheese, or herbs to create a flavor profile that suits your taste buds.

By including protein-packed breakfasts featuring eggs in your meal rotation, you can enjoy the benefits of high-quality protein, improved satiety, and a wide range of essential nutrients. The chapter will provide you with inspiration and ideas for incorporating eggs into your breakfast routine, allowing you to create delicious and nutritious meals to support your weight loss goals and overall well-being.

Egg-based recipes for protein-rich breakfasts

Eggs are a versatile ingredient that can be used to create a wide range of protein-rich breakfast options. In this section, we will delve into various egg-based recipes, highlighting their protein content and providing readers with delicious and nutritious meal ideas. Here are a few popular egg-based recipes:

Omelets: Omelets are a classic breakfast choice that allows for endless customization. Start with whisked eggs and add your choice of vegetables, such as spinach, bell peppers, onions, or mushrooms. You can also include lean proteins like diced chicken or turkey, or incorporate cheese for added flavor and protein.

Frittatas: Frittatas are oven-baked egg dishes that are incredibly versatile. They can be made with various ingredients, such as diced vegetables, herbs, and cheeses. Frittatas can be a great option for meal prepping, as they can be made in advance and enjoyed throughout the week.

Egg Muffins: Egg muffins are portable and convenient protein-packed breakfast options. They are made by whisking eggs with your desired ingredients, such as chopped vegetables, cooked bacon or sausage, and cheese. Pour the mixture into muffin tins and bake until set. Egg muffins can be made ahead of time and stored in the refrigerator for a quick and easy grab-and-go breakfast.

Shakshuka: Shakshuka is a popular Middle Eastern dish made by simmering eggs in a tomato-based sauce with onions, bell peppers, and spices. It's a flavorful and protein-rich option that can be enjoyed for breakfast or brunch.

Egg Wraps: Replace traditional tortillas with thin omelets to create protein-packed wraps. Fill the omelet with ingredients like sliced avocado, turkey or chicken slices, lettuce, and tomatoes. Roll it up and enjoy a nutritious and satisfying breakfast.

Egg Salad: Hard-boiled eggs can be used to create a protein-rich egg salad. Chop boiled eggs and mix them with Greek yogurt or mayonnaise, diced celery or pickles, mustard, and seasonings. Serve it on whole grain bread or lettuce wraps for a filling breakfast option.

Scrambled Eggs: Scrambled eggs are a simple and quick option that can be customized with various add-ins. Incorporate vegetables like spinach, tomatoes, or mushrooms, and add a sprinkle of cheese or herbs for extra flavor.

Breakfast Burritos: Fill tortillas with scrambled eggs, black beans, diced vegetables, and a dollop of Greek yogurt or salsa. Roll them up and enjoy a protein-packed breakfast on the go.

Spinach and Feta Omelet: Whisk together eggs, and pour them into a heated non-stick skillet. Add sautéed spinach and crumbled feta cheese to one side of the omelet. Fold the other side over the filling and cook until the cheese is melted. Serve with a side of whole grain toast.

Veggie Egg Muffins: Preheat the oven and whisk together eggs and a splash of milk in a bowl. Add diced vegetables like bell peppers, onions, and broccoli to the egg mixture. Pour the mixture into a greased muffin tin and bake until set. Enjoy these protein-packed egg muffins as a grab-and-go breakfast option.

Smoked Salmon Scrambled Eggs: Whisk eggs with a bit of cream or milk in a bowl. In a non-stick skillet, melt butter and add beaten eggs. Stir in slices of smoked salmon and cook until the eggs are fluffy and cooked to your liking. Season with salt, pepper, and fresh herbs for added flavor.

Bacon and Cheddar Frittata: Cook bacon until crispy, then crumble it. In a bowl, whisk together eggs, milk, and shredded cheddar cheese. Pour the mixture into a greased oven-safe skillet and sprinkle the crumbled bacon on top. Bake until the frittata is set and golden brown. Serve with a side salad for a satisfying breakfast.

Southwest Breakfast Burrito: Scramble eggs with diced bell peppers, onions, and black beans. Warm tortillas and fill them with the scrambled egg mixture. Top with salsa, avocado slices, and a sprinkle of shredded cheese. Roll up the burrito and enjoy a protein-packed breakfast on the go.

Mushroom and Goat Cheese Omelet: Sauté sliced mushrooms in a skillet until tender. In a separate bowl, whisk together eggs and crumbled goat cheese. Pour the egg mixture into the skillet with the mushrooms and cook until set. Fold the omelet over the filling and serve with a side of whole grain toast.

Caprese Egg Cups: Line a muffin tin with slices of ham or turkey, creating a cup shape. Crack an egg into each ham cup and top with a slice of tomato and a sprinkle of mozzarella cheese. Bake until the eggs are cooked to your liking. These delicious egg cups are a protein-packed breakfast option.

Remember, the beauty of egg-based recipes is their versatility. Feel free to experiment with different ingredients, spices, and seasonings to create a variety of protein-rich breakfast options that suit your taste preferences and dietary needs.

Vegetarian alternatives using tofu or legumes

For individuals following a vegetarian diet or looking for meatless alternatives, tofu and legumes can be excellent sources of protein in egg-based breakfast recipes. Here are some vegetarian alternatives that incorporate tofu or legumes.

Tofu Scramble: Replace eggs with crumbled tofu in a scramble recipe. Sauté tofu in a skillet with your choice of vegetables, such as bell peppers, onions, and spinach. Season with turmeric, cumin, and nutritional yeast for a flavorful and protein-packed breakfast option.

Chickpea Flour Omelet: Instead of using eggs, make an omelet using chickpea flour (also known as besan or gram flour). Whisk chickpea flour with water and seasonings like salt, pepper, and herbs. Cook the batter in a non-stick skillet with your preferred fillings, such as sautéed vegetables and vegan cheese.

Lentil Breakfast Bowl: Cook lentils and toss them with sautéed vegetables like kale, cherry tomatoes, and mushrooms.

Add your favorite spices and herbs, such as garlic, paprika, and fresh cilantro. Serve the lentil mixture as a hearty and protein-rich breakfast bowl.

Black Bean Breakfast Burrito: Replace eggs with mashed black beans in a breakfast burrito. Spread a layer of black beans on a tortilla and top with diced avocado, salsa, and a sprinkle of vegan cheese. Roll it up and enjoy a flavorful and protein-packed breakfast wrap.

Tofu and Vegetable Frittata: Use crumbled tofu instead of eggs in a frittata recipe. Sauté tofu with diced vegetables like zucchini, bell peppers, and onions. Season with spices like turmeric, garlic powder, and nutritional yeast. Bake until the frittata is set and golden brown.

Chickpea Pancakes: Make savory pancakes using chickpea flour and water. Mix chickpea flour with water, salt, and spices like cumin and paprika. Cook the batter like regular pancakes and serve with toppings like avocado, cherry tomatoes, and a drizzle of tahini sauce.

Tofu Breakfast Burrito: Crumble tofu and sauté it with diced vegetables, such as bell peppers, onions, and spinach. Add spices like chili powder, cumin, and garlic powder for flavor. Fill a tortilla with the tofu mixture and top with salsa and sliced avocado.

These vegetarian alternatives provide a great source of plant-based protein, offering a tasty and nutritious start to your day. Feel free to experiment with different flavors and ingredients to customize these recipes to your liking.

Incorporating vegetables and herbs for added flavor and nutrients

Incorporating vegetables and herbs into your egg-based breakfast recipes not only adds flavor but also boosts the nutritional value of your meal. Here are some ways to include vegetables and herbs for added taste and nutrients.

Sautéed Vegetable Omelet: Dice and sauté a variety of vegetables like bell peppers, onions, mushrooms, and spinach. Add the sautéed vegetables as a filling in your omelet, along with cheese or other desired ingredients.

The vegetables add texture, flavor, and an array of vitamins and minerals.

Garden Veggie Scramble: Chop vegetables such as zucchini, tomatoes, broccoli, and asparagus into small pieces. Sauté them in a skillet with a little olive oil or cooking spray until tender. Add beaten eggs and scramble together, seasoning with herbs like basil, thyme, or parsley for an extra burst of flavor.

Mediterranean Frittata: Combine diced tomatoes, chopped spinach, sliced olives, and crumbled feta cheese in a bowl. Pour the mixture into a greased oven-safe skillet and pour beaten eggs over the top. Bake until set and garnish with fresh herbs like oregano or dill for a Mediterranean-inspired breakfast.

Herb and Mushroom Egg Muffins: Sauté sliced mushrooms and fresh herbs such as rosemary or thyme in a skillet until tender. Mix them into beaten eggs along with some shredded cheese. Pour the mixture into greased muffin cups and bake until set. These savory egg muffins are packed with flavor and nutrients.

Green Goddess Scramble: Blend leafy greens like spinach, kale, or Swiss chard with eggs and a splash of milk or plant-based milk. Cook the mixture in a skillet until scrambled and add fresh herbs like cilantro, basil, or mint for a vibrant and nutritious green scramble.

Tomato and Basil Egg Cups: Line muffin cups with slices of tomato and sprinkle fresh basil leaves on top. Crack an egg into each cup and bake until the eggs are set. The combination of juicy tomatoes and aromatic basil gives these egg cups a burst of freshness.

Herb-infused Egg Salad: Make a protein-rich egg salad by combining hard-boiled eggs with diced celery, red onion, and fresh herbs like dill or chives. Season with salt, pepper, and a squeeze of lemon juice. Enjoy the egg salad on whole grain bread or as a topping for salads.

By incorporating vegetables and herbs into your egg-based breakfasts, you enhance the flavor profile, add essential nutrients, and increase the overall healthfulness of your meal. Experiment with different combinations and herbs to create exciting and delicious breakfast options.

Chapter 6: The Power of Plant-Based Breakfasts: Nourishment from Nature

As plant-based diets gain increasing popularity, it's important to explore the benefits they offer for overall health and well-being. This chapter delves into the growing popularity and benefits of plant-based diets, specifically focusing on plant-based breakfasts and their impact on our health. Here are some key points to consider.

Rising Popularity: Plant-based diets, which emphasize whole plant foods while minimizing or excluding animal products, have gained traction in recent years. Many individuals are adopting plant-based lifestyles due to ethical, environmental, and health reasons. The shift towards plant-based eating is fueled by a growing awareness of the potential benefits it offers.

Health Benefits: Plant-based diets have been associated with numerous health benefits. They tend to be rich in fiber, vitamins, minerals, and phytochemicals while being lower in saturated fat and cholesterol compared to traditional Western diets. Research suggests that plant-based diets can help prevent and manage chronic diseases such as heart disease, type 2 diabetes, obesity, and certain types of cancer.

Nutrient Density: Plant-based breakfasts allow individuals to start their day with a wide variety of nutrient-dense foods. Fruits, vegetables, whole grains, legumes, nuts, and seeds provide essential vitamins, minerals, antioxidants, and dietary fiber. These plant foods offer a spectrum of nutrients that support optimal health and well-being.

Increased Fiber Intake: Plant-based breakfasts are typically high in dietary fiber, which has numerous health benefits. Fiber aids digestion, promotes satiety, helps maintain a healthy weight, and supports a healthy gut microbiome. By starting the day with fiber-rich plant foods, individuals can enhance their digestive health and promote a feeling of fullness, reducing the likelihood of overeating later in the day.

Reduced Environmental Impact: Plant-based diets have a lower environmental footprint compared to diets centered around animal products. Livestock farming contributes to greenhouse gas emissions, deforestation, and water pollution. By choosing plant-based breakfasts, individuals can contribute to a more sustainable and eco-friendly food system.

Versatility and Creativity: Plant-based breakfasts offer endless possibilities for creating delicious and satisfying meals. From smoothie bowls and overnight oats to avocado toasts and tofu scrambles, plant-based options are versatile and allow individuals to explore new flavors and textures. This flexibility ensures that plant-based breakfasts can be enjoyable, nourishing, and tailored to individual tastes.

Supporting Ethical Considerations: Plant-based diets align with ethical considerations related to animal welfare. By choosing plant-based breakfasts, individuals can support a more compassionate and humane approach to food consumption, reducing the demand for animal products and their associated ethical concerns.

Overall, the growing popularity of plant-based diets stems from their potential health benefits, environmental sustainability, and ethical considerations. Plant-based breakfasts provide a nourishing and delicious way to kick-start the day while supporting overall health and well-being. In the following sections of this chapter, we will explore a wide range of plant-based breakfast options that showcase the power of plant-based eating.

Incorporating plant-based foods into breakfast is an essential step towards a nutritious and satisfying start to the day. Plant-based breakfasts offer a wide range of health benefits, including increased nutrient intake, improved digestion, sustainable weight management, and reduced risk of chronic diseases. Let's delve into the importance of incorporating plant-based foods into breakfast in more detail.

Nutrient Density: Plant-based foods, such as fruits, vegetables, whole grains, legumes, nuts, and seeds, are rich in essential vitamins, minerals, antioxidants, and dietary fiber. By including these nutrient-dense foods in our breakfast, we ensure that our bodies receive the necessary nourishment to support optimal health and well-being.

Fiber-Rich Start: Plant-based breakfasts are typically high in dietary fiber, which offers numerous health benefits. Fiber aids in digestion, promotes satiety, regulates blood sugar levels, and supports a healthy gut microbiome. Starting the day with fiber-rich foods like whole grains, fruits, and vegetables helps maintain a healthy digestive system and provides a feeling of fullness, preventing overeating later in the day.

Sustainable Weight Management: Plant-based breakfasts, with their high fiber and nutrient content, can contribute to sustainable weight management. The fiber and water content in plant-based foods promote a feeling of fullness, reducing the likelihood of overeating and aiding in weight control. Additionally, plant-based diets tend to be lower in calorie density and saturated fats, which can further support weight management efforts.

Disease Prevention: Research suggests that plant-based diets can help prevent and manage chronic diseases, including heart disease, type 2 diabetes, obesity, and certain types of cancer. The abundance of antioxidants and phytochemicals found in plant-based foods helps combat inflammation and oxidative stress, which are underlying factors in the development of many chronic diseases.

Environmental Considerations: Incorporating plant-based foods into breakfast aligns with sustainable and eco-friendly practices. Animal agriculture has a significant environmental impact, contributing to greenhouse gas emissions, deforestation, and water pollution. By choosing plant-based options, we reduce our ecological footprint and support a more sustainable food system.

Culinary Versatility: Plant-based breakfasts offer a wide range of culinary possibilities and flavors. From smoothie bowls and overnight oats to vegetable scrambles and plant-based protein sources like tofu or tempeh, there are endless options to explore. Incorporating plant-based foods into breakfast allows for creativity and culinary adventure while providing nourishment and satisfaction.

Vital Antioxidants: Plant-based foods are abundant in antioxidants, which help protect the body against oxidative stress and inflammation. Antioxidants play a vital role in supporting immune function, reducing the risk of chronic diseases, and promoting cellular health. Breakfast is an excellent opportunity to incorporate antioxidant-rich foods like berries, leafy greens, and colorful fruits.

Sustainable and Eco-Friendly: Plant-based breakfasts contribute to a more sustainable and eco-friendly food system. By reducing the reliance on animal products, you decrease your environmental impact, including greenhouse gas emissions, water usage, and deforestation. Choosing plant-based options helps support a healthier planet for future generations.

Variety and Flavor: Plant-based breakfasts offer a wide range of flavors, textures, and culinary creativity. From smoothie bowls to grain-based breakfast bowls, savory tofu scrambles to veggie-packed omelets, there are endless possibilities to explore. Incorporating plant-based foods into your breakfast allows you to experiment with different ingredients and expand your palate.

Weight Management and Energy Levels: Plant-based breakfasts can support weight management goals by providing nutrient-dense, low-calorie options that promote feelings of fullness. The fiber and protein content in plant-based foods help regulate appetite, prevent overeating, and maintain energy levels throughout the morning.

Mindful and Conscious Eating: Plant-based breakfasts encourage mindful and conscious eating. By choosing whole, unprocessed foods, you become more aware of the ingredients you consume and their impact on your health. This mindfulness fosters a positive relationship with food and can lead to better food choices throughout the day.

The abundance of nutrients, fiber, and antioxidants found in plant-based ingredients forms the foundation of a healthy and nourishing diet.

Incorporating plant-based ingredients into your meals, especially breakfast, provides an array of essential nutrients, fiber, and antioxidants that promote optimal health and well-being. By embracing the abundance of plant-based foods, you can enjoy delicious and satisfying meals while reaping the benefits of their nutrient density and disease-fighting properties.

Plant-based breakfast options for vegans and vegetarians

For vegans and vegetarians, adopting a plant-based lifestyle extends beyond excluding animal products. It involves embracing a wide range of nutrient-rich plant foods to ensure a balanced and satisfying breakfast. This section explores a variety of plant-based breakfast options tailored specifically for vegans and vegetarians. Here are some delicious and nourishing plant-based breakfast ideas:

Smoothie Bowls: Start your day with a vibrant and nutrient-packed smoothie bowl. Blend together frozen fruits, such as berries or tropical fruits, with a plant-based milk or yogurt, and add a handful of leafy greens for an extra nutritional boost. Top it with sliced fruits, nuts, seeds, and granola for added texture and flavor.

Overnight Chia Pudding: Combine chia seeds with your choice of plant-based milk, sweetener, and flavorings like vanilla or cocoa powder. Mix well and let it sit in the refrigerator overnight. In the morning, top it with fresh fruits, nuts, and seeds for a creamy and filling breakfast.

Avocado Toast: Spread mashed avocado on whole grain toast and add toppings like sliced tomatoes, sprouts, and a sprinkle of sea salt and black pepper. Enhance the flavor with a squeeze of lemon juice or a drizzle of balsamic glaze.

Tofu Scramble: Create a delicious and protein-packed tofu scramble by crumbling firm tofu and sautéing it with vegetables like bell peppers, onions, and spinach. Season it with spices like turmeric, cumin, and paprika for a savory and satisfying breakfast.

Veggie Breakfast Burrito: Wrap scrambled tofu or sautéed vegetables in a whole grain tortilla for a portable and nutritious breakfast. Add toppings like avocado, salsa, and vegan cheese for extra flavor.

Quinoa Breakfast Bowl: Cook quinoa in plant-based milk, and sweeten it with maple syrup or agave. Top it with sliced fruits, nuts, and a sprinkle of cinnamon for a protein-packed and fiber-rich breakfast.

Chickpea Pancakes: Make savory chickpea pancakes by blending chickpea flour, water, and spices like garlic powder, cumin, and paprika. Cook the batter on a griddle and serve with a side of avocado or tomato salsa.

Lentil Breakfast Bowl: Cook lentils until tender and toss them with roasted vegetables, fresh herbs, and a drizzle of olive oil. Add a squeeze of lemon juice for a tangy kick and enjoy a hearty and satisfying breakfast bowl.

Vegan Breakfast Burrito Bowl: Create a breakfast bowl with a base of cooked quinoa or brown rice. Top it with black beans, sautéed vegetables, avocado slices, and a dollop of vegan sour cream or salsa for a flavorful and filling meal.

Nut Butter and Fruit Wrap: Spread your favorite nut butter on a whole grain tortilla and top it with sliced fruits like bananas or berries. Roll it up and enjoy a delicious and portable plant-based breakfast.

Vegan Protein Pancakes: Make fluffy and protein-rich pancakes using a combination of plant-based protein powder, mashed bananas, oat flour, and plant-based milk. Serve them with a drizzle of pure maple syrup and a sprinkle of nuts or seeds for added crunch.

Green Smoothie Bowl: Blend together a mix of leafy greens, like spinach or kale, with a frozen banana, plant-based milk, and a scoop of nut butter. Pour the smoothie into a bowl and top it with sliced fruits, coconut flakes, and a handful of granola for a refreshing and nutrient-packed breakfast.

Vegan Breakfast Sausages: Prepare delicious and meat-free breakfast sausages using ingredients like tempeh or textured vegetable protein. Season them with herbs and spices, then pan-fry or bake until crispy. Serve them alongside whole grain toast or in a breakfast sandwich for a protein-packed start to your day.

Vegan Yogurt Parfait: Layer plant-based yogurt with a mixture of fresh fruits, nuts, and seeds in a glass or jar. Add a drizzle of agave or a sprinkle of cinnamon for a tasty and satisfying breakfast parfait.

Vegan Breakfast Casserole: Create a savory breakfast casserole using ingredients like tofu, vegetables, and vegan cheese. Bake it until golden and serve it as a filling and flavorful breakfast option for weekends or special occasions.

Vegan Breakfast Burrito with Tofu: Wrap scrambled tofu, sautéed vegetables, and black beans in a whole grain tortilla. Add a dollop of vegan sour cream or salsa for a satisfying and portable breakfast on the go.

Vegan Breakfast Hash: Sauté diced potatoes, bell peppers, onions, and vegan sausage in a skillet until golden and crispy. Season it with herbs and spices like paprika, garlic powder, and thyme for a delicious and hearty plant-based breakfast hash.

Vegan Quiche: Create a plant-based quiche using a tofu-based filling mixed with vegetables, herbs, and spices. Bake it in a pie crust made from whole grain flour for a savory and protein-packed breakfast option.

Vegan Breakfast Sandwich: Assemble a hearty breakfast sandwich using whole grain bread, vegan cheese, avocado slices, and tempeh bacon or grilled vegetables. Add some greens and a spread of vegan mayo or mustard for a satisfying and flavorful morning meal.

Vegan Protein Oatmeal: Cook oats in plant-based milk and add a scoop of your favorite vegan protein powder. Sweeten it with natural sweeteners like maple syrup or dates, and top it with fruits, nuts, and seeds for a protein-rich and filling breakfast.

These plant-based breakfast options for vegans and vegetarians are not only delicious but also provide essential nutrients like protein, fiber, vitamins, and minerals. By incorporating a variety of plant-based foods into their morning routine, individuals can enjoy a nutritious and satisfying breakfast that supports their health and aligns with their dietary choices.

Benefits of plant-based proteins

Plant-based proteins offer numerous benefits for overall health and well-being. They are derived from sources such as legumes, grains, nuts, seeds, and vegetables, and are typically low in saturated fat and cholesterol. Plant-based proteins are rich in fiber, vitamins, minerals, and antioxidants, making them an excellent choice for individuals following a vegetarian or vegan diet, as well as those looking to incorporate more plant-based foods into their meals. Here are some benefits of plant-based proteins:

Heart Health: Plant-based proteins are typically low in saturated fat and cholesterol, which can help maintain healthy cholesterol levels and reduce the risk of heart disease.

Weight Management: Plant-based proteins are often lower in calories and higher in fiber, promoting satiety and aiding in weight management.

Reduced Inflammation: Plant-based proteins are associated with anti-inflammatory properties, which can help reduce chronic inflammation in the body and lower the risk of inflammatory diseases.

Improved Digestion: The high fiber content in plant-based proteins can support healthy digestion and prevent constipation.

Blood Sugar Control: Plant-based proteins have a lower glycemic index compared to animal-based proteins, helping to regulate blood sugar levels and manage diabetes.

Lower Risk of Chronic Diseases: A diet rich in plant-based proteins has been linked to a reduced risk of chronic conditions, including type 2 diabetes, certain types of cancer, and cardiovascular diseases.

Nutrient-Dense: Plant-based proteins are packed with essential nutrients like vitamins, minerals, and antioxidants that support overall health and vitality.

Sustainability: Plant-based proteins have a lower environmental impact compared to animal-based proteins, making them a more sustainable choice for the planet.

Improved Gut Health: The fiber content in plant-based proteins acts as a prebiotic, promoting the growth of beneficial gut bacteria and supporting a healthy gut microbiome.

Anti-Aging Properties: Plant-based proteins contain antioxidants that help fight free radicals and protect against oxidative stress, which can contribute to aging and age-related diseases.

Balanced pH Levels: Plant-based proteins have an alkalizing effect on the body, helping to maintain a balanced pH level and prevent chronic acidity.

Enhanced Athletic Performance: Plant-based proteins can provide the necessary amino acids for muscle repair and recovery, supporting athletic performance and muscle growth.

Bone Health: Plant-based proteins often contain calcium and other bone-building nutrients, contributing to optimal bone health and reducing the risk of osteoporosis.

Improved Skin Health: The antioxidants found in plant-based proteins can promote healthy skin by protecting against damage from environmental factors and promoting collagen production.

Reduced Allergy Risk: Plant-based proteins are less likely to cause allergic reactions compared to animal-based proteins, making them a suitable choice for individuals with food allergies or sensitivities.

Lower Environmental Impact: Plant-based proteins require fewer resources, such as land and water, to produce, reducing their environmental footprint compared to animal-based proteins.

Longevity: Studies have shown that individuals following a plant-based diet have a longer life expectancy and a lower risk of premature death.

Boosted Immune Function: Plant-based proteins provide essential vitamins and minerals that support a healthy immune system and help fight off infections and diseases.

Sustainable Weight Loss: Plant-based proteins can contribute to sustainable weight loss by providing nutrients, promoting satiety, and reducing cravings for unhealthy foods.

Ethical Considerations: Plant-based proteins align with ethical considerations such as animal welfare, making them a compassionate choice for individuals who prioritize animal rights.

These benefits highlight the advantages of incorporating plant-based proteins into a balanced and varied diet, supporting overall health, sustainability, and a mindful approach to nutrition.

Unique plant-based breakfast ideas and recipes

Plant-based breakfasts offer a wide range of delicious and creative options that are both nutritious and satisfying. Here are some unique plant-based breakfast ideas and recipes to inspire your morning meals:

Chia Seed Pudding: Combine chia seeds with your choice of plant-based milk, sweetener, and flavorings like vanilla or cocoa powder. Let it sit overnight for a creamy and nutrient-packed pudding. Top with fresh fruits, nuts, and seeds.

Avocado Toast: Mash ripe avocado onto whole grain toast and sprinkle with sea salt, black pepper, and a squeeze of lemon juice. Customize with additional toppings such as sliced tomatoes, microgreens, or a drizzle of balsamic glaze.

Vegetable Hash: Sauté a medley of colorful vegetables like bell peppers, onions, zucchini, and sweet potatoes in a bit of olive oil. Season with herbs and spices like paprika, cumin, and thyme for a flavorful and hearty breakfast option.

Tofu Scramble: Crumble firm tofu and sauté with a variety of vegetables, such as bell peppers, spinach, mushrooms, and onions. Season with turmeric, nutritional yeast, garlic powder, and soy sauce for a savory and protein-packed scramble.

Breakfast Quinoa Bowl: Cook quinoa and top it with your favorite plant-based milk, fresh fruits, nuts, and a drizzle of maple syrup or honey. Add a sprinkle of cinnamon for extra flavor.

Vegan Pancakes: Make fluffy pancakes using a combination of mashed bananas, plant-based milk, whole wheat flour, and baking powder. Serve with fruit compote, nut butter, or a dollop of coconut yogurt.

Sweet Potato Toast: Slice sweet potatoes into thin rounds and toast until tender. Top with nut butter, sliced bananas, and a sprinkle of cinnamon, or try savory toppings like avocado, hummus, and sprouts.

Smoothie Bowl: Blend a thick smoothie using your choice of plant-based milk, frozen fruits, and leafy greens. Pour into a bowl and top with granola, sliced fruits, coconut flakes, and chia seeds for a refreshing and nutrient-dense breakfast.

Veggie Breakfast Burrito: Fill a whole grain tortilla with scrambled tofu or black beans, sautéed vegetables, salsa, and avocado. Roll it up and enjoy a protein-packed and satisfying breakfast on the go.

Overnight Oats: Combine rolled oats with your choice of plant-based milk, chia seeds, and a sweetener like maple syrup or agave. Let it sit overnight in the fridge, and in the morning, top with fresh fruits, nuts, and a drizzle of nut butter.

Banana Bread Protein Muffins: Make homemade banana bread muffins using whole wheat flour, mashed bananas, plant-based protein powder, and a touch of sweetness from dates or maple syrup.

Green Smoothie Pancakes: Blend spinach or kale with plant-based milk, banana, oats, and a touch of baking powder to create a vibrant and nutritious pancake batter. Cook them on a griddle and serve with fresh berries and a dollop of coconut yogurt.

Coconut Chia Pudding Parfait: Layer coconut chia pudding with mixed berries, granola, and a sprinkle of shredded coconut for a tropical and satisfying breakfast parfait.

Quinoa Breakfast Cookies: Combine cooked quinoa with mashed bananas, nut butter, nuts, dried fruits, and a touch of sweetener. Shape into cookies and bake for a delicious and protein-rich breakfast treat.

Lentil Breakfast Bowl: Cook lentils and serve them with roasted vegetables, a dollop of tahini, and a sprinkle of fresh herbs like parsley or cilantro. Add a squeeze of lemon juice for a bright and flavorful breakfast bowl.

Peanut Butter and Jelly Oat Bars: Make homemade oat bars using oats, peanut butter, chia seeds, and a layer of your favorite fruit jam. These portable bars are perfect for a quick and nutritious breakfast on the go.

Veggie Frittata: Whisk together chickpea flour, plant-based milk, and spices like turmeric, garlic powder, and nutritional yeast. Add a variety of sautéed vegetables and bake until set for a protein-rich and flavorful frittata.

Mexican Breakfast Bowl: Top cooked quinoa or brown rice with black beans, salsa, avocado slices, and a sprinkle of nutritional yeast or vegan cheese for a satisfying and Mexican-inspired breakfast.

Mango Coconut Chia Pudding Parfait: Layer chia pudding made with coconut milk, fresh mango slices, and toasted coconut flakes for a tropical and creamy breakfast parfait.

Spirulina Smoothie Bowl: Blend frozen bananas, plant-based milk, and a teaspoon of spirulina powder for a vibrant and nutrient-packed smoothie bowl. Top with sliced fruits, granola, and hemp seeds for added crunch and nutrition.

These plant-based breakfast ideas and recipes provide a variety of flavors, textures, and nutrients to help you start your day off right while enjoying the benefits of a plant-based lifestyle. Feel free to customize and experiment with different ingredients to suit your taste preferences and dietary needs.

Chapter 7: Creative Grab-and-Go Options: Breakfast on the Run

In today's fast-paced world, many individuals find themselves rushing in the morning, often sacrificing a nutritious breakfast. However, with a little planning and preparation, it is possible to enjoy a healthy breakfast even on the busiest of days. This Chapter is dedicated to providing practical and delicious breakfast ideas that can be easily prepared ahead of time and enjoyed on the go.

This chapter aims to address the common challenge of time constraints by offering convenient and portable breakfast options that do not compromise on nutrition. It emphasizes the importance of fueling your body with wholesome ingredients to kickstart your day and maintain energy levels.

You will discover a variety of make-ahead breakfast ideas that can be prepared in advance, allowing you to grab a nutritious meal on your way out the door. These options are designed to be portable, mess-free, and easily consumed during commutes, at the office, or wherever your busy schedule takes you.

The chapter will provide guidance on planning and prepping breakfasts ahead of time, including tips for batch cooking, proper storage, and selecting the right containers to maintain freshness. It will also offer suggestions for balancing macronutrients, such as incorporating a mix of proteins, whole grains, and fruits or vegetables for a well-rounded meal.

In addition to practical tips, this chapter will highlight the importance of mindful eating, even when on the go. It will encourage readers to take a moment to savor and enjoy their breakfast, even in a fast-paced environment, to promote better digestion and overall well-being.

By the end of this chapter, you will be equipped with a repertoire of delicious and nutritious grab-and-go breakfast options that suit their lifestyle. You'll will have the knowledge and confidence to make healthier choices when pressed for time, ensuring that they start their day off right with a balanced and satisfying meal.

Whether you're a busy professional, a student rushing to class, or a parent juggling multiple responsibilities, Chapter 7 will empower you to prioritize your health and nourish your body with quick and convenient breakfast options that support your weight loss journey.

Quick and convenient breakfast ideas for busy individuals

In today's fast-paced world, busy individuals often find themselves struggling to make time for a nutritious breakfast. However, skipping breakfast can lead to decreased energy levels, poor concentration, and cravings for unhealthy foods throughout the day. As a registered dietitian, I understand the challenges faced by individuals striving to maintain a healthy lifestyle amidst their hectic schedules. That's why I have compiled a collection of quick and convenient breakfast ideas that will help nourish your body and set you up for success, even on the busiest of mornings.

Overnight Chia Pudding:
Prepare a delicious and satisfying breakfast the night before by combining chia seeds with your choice of plant-based milk, such as almond or coconut milk. Add a touch of sweetness with a natural sweetener like maple syrup or honey. Let it sit in the refrigerator overnight, and in the morning, top it with fresh fruits, nuts, and a sprinkle of cinnamon for a nutrient-packed breakfast that requires no cooking.

Nut Butter and Banana Wrap:
Grab a whole-grain tortilla and spread a generous amount of your favorite nut butter, such as almond or peanut butter. Place a ripe banana in the center and roll it up into a wrap. This simple yet delicious option provides a balance of carbohydrates, healthy fats, and natural sugars to fuel your morning.

Greek Yogurt Parfait:
Layer Greek yogurt with a variety of toppings, such as fresh berries, granola, and a drizzle of honey. Greek yogurt is rich in protein, which will help keep you satisfied and energized throughout the day. The combination of textures and flavors in this parfait makes it a delightful and nutritious option.

Veggie Egg Muffins:
Prepare a batch of veggie egg muffins ahead of time by whisking together eggs, chopped vegetables, and your favorite herbs and spices. Pour the mixture into muffin tins and bake until set. These portable and protein-packed muffins can be stored in the refrigerator and reheated in the morning for a quick and filling breakfast.

Smoothie on the Go:
Blend together a combination of frozen fruits, leafy greens, your choice of milk or yogurt, and a scoop of protein powder. Pour the smoothie into a portable container and take it with you on your morning commute. Smoothies are a convenient way to pack in a variety of nutrients, and they can be customized to your taste preferences.

Overnight Oats:

Combine rolled oats, your choice of milk, and toppings such as nuts, seeds, and dried fruits in a jar or container. Let it sit overnight in the refrigerator, and in the morning, you'll have a ready-to-eat breakfast that can be enjoyed cold or warmed up. Overnight oats are not only quick and easy but also provide a good source of fiber and complex carbohydrates.

Portable Breakfast Bars:

Make a batch of homemade breakfast bars using wholesome ingredients like oats, nuts, seeds, and dried fruits. These bars can be prepared in advance and stored in individual portions for a grab-and-go breakfast option. Look for recipes that use natural sweeteners like dates or honey to keep added sugars to a minimum.

Avocado Toast:
Toast a slice of whole-grain bread and top it with mashed avocado, a sprinkle of sea salt, and a squeeze of lemon or lime juice. For an extra boost of nutrients, add toppings like sliced tomatoes, cucumber, or a poached egg. Avocado toast provides healthy fats, fiber, and a variety of vitamins and minerals to start your day off right.

Protein Pancakes:
Whisk together a combination of whole-grain flour, protein powder, and your choice of milk to create a protein-rich pancake batter. Cook the pancakes on a non-stick skillet until golden brown. Serve them with a drizzle of pure maple syrup or a dollop

of Greek yogurt and fresh berries. These fluffy pancakes provide a satisfying and nutrient-packed breakfast option.

Breakfast Burrito:
Fill a whole-grain tortilla with scrambled eggs or tofu, sautéed vegetables, and a sprinkle of cheese. Add a touch of hot sauce or salsa for extra flavor. Roll it up and wrap it in foil for a portable and satisfying breakfast that you can enjoy on the go.

Fruit and Yogurt Bowl:
Start with a base of Greek yogurt or dairy-free yogurt alternative. Top it with a variety of fresh fruits, such as berries, sliced bananas, or diced mango. Sprinkle some nuts, seeds, or granola on top for added crunch and nutrition. This vibrant and refreshing bowl is

packed with vitamins, minerals, and antioxidants to kick-start your day.

Quinoa Breakfast Bowl:
Cook quinoa according to package instructions and top it with a combination of sliced almonds, dried fruits, and a drizzle of honey or pure maple syrup. You can also add a splash of plant-based milk for added creaminess. Quinoa is a complete protein and a great source of fiber, making it a nutritious and filling breakfast option.

Energy Balls:
Prepare a batch of homemade energy balls using a mixture of nuts, seeds, dried fruits, and a binder like nut butter or dates. These bite-sized treats are packed with energy-boosting nutrients and can be easily stored in the

refrigerator for quick and convenient breakfast options throughout the week.

Veggie Breakfast Wrap:
Wrap scrambled eggs or tofu, sautéed vegetables, and a sprinkle of cheese in a whole-grain tortilla. Add some avocado slices or a dollop of salsa for extra flavor. This savory breakfast wrap provides a good balance of protein, fiber, and essential nutrients to keep you satisfied until your next meal.

Cottage Cheese Delight:
Combine cottage cheese with a variety of toppings, such as sliced fresh fruits, nuts, and a drizzle of honey. Cottage cheese is rich in protein and calcium, making it a nutritious and filling option for a busy morning.

Breakfast Quiche Cups:

Prepare mini quiche cups using a muffin tin. Whisk together eggs, chopped vegetables, and your choice of cheese. Pour the mixture into the muffin tin and bake until set. These mini quiches are portable, customizable, and can be enjoyed warm or cold.

Breakfast Trail Mix:
Create your own custom trail mix using a combination of nuts, dried fruits, seeds, and whole-grain cereal. Pack it in individual portions or small containers for a quick and easy breakfast option that you can munch on throughout the morning.

Savory Oatmeal Bowl:
Instead of the traditional sweet oatmeal, prepare a savory version by

cooking oats in vegetable broth or water and topping them with sautéed vegetables, a poached egg or tofu, and a sprinkle of herbs and spices. This savory twist on oatmeal provides a nourishing and filling breakfast option.

Breakfast Quesadilla:
Fill a whole-grain tortilla with scrambled eggs or tofu, chopped vegetables, and a sprinkle of cheese. Cook it on a skillet until the tortilla is crispy and the filling is warmed through. Cut it into wedges and serve it with salsa or Greek yogurt for dipping.

Green Smoothie Bowl:
Blend together a combination of leafy greens, frozen fruits, and your choice of milk or yogurt to create a thick and creamy smoothie. Pour the smoothie into a bowl and top it with nutritious

toppings such as sliced fresh fruits, nuts, seeds, and a sprinkle of granola or coconut flakes. This vibrant and nutrient-dense bowl not only provides a refreshing start to your day but also ensures you get a good dose of vitamins, minerals, and antioxidants.

With these quick and convenient breakfast ideas, busy individuals can fuel their bodies with nourishing meals even on the busiest of mornings. By prioritizing a nutritious breakfast, you set the foundation for a productive and energized day ahead. Remember to choose options that are rich in protein, fiber, and essential nutrients to keep you satisfied and fueled until your next meal. With a little planning and creativity, you can enjoy delicious and wholesome breakfasts that support your overall health and well-being.

Start your day off right with these hassle-free breakfast options and embrace the benefits of nourishing your body on the go.

The time required to prepare the breakfasts mentioned can vary depending on the recipe and individual cooking skills. Here is a general estimate of the preparation time for each breakfast idea.

Overnight Chia Pudding: 5 minutes of active preparation time + overnight soaking.

Smoothie: 5 minutes or less, depending on the ingredients and blender used.

Protein Pancakes: 10-15 minutes, including mixing the batter and cooking time.

Breakfast Burrito: 10-15 minutes, depending on the filling preparation and assembly.

Fruit and Yogurt Bowl: 5 minutes or less, depending on the fruit chopping and topping selection.

Quinoa Breakfast Bowl: 15-20 minutes, including cooking the quinoa and assembling the toppings.

Energy Balls: 15-20 minutes, including mixing the ingredients and shaping the balls.

Veggie Breakfast Wrap: 10-15 minutes, including preparing the fillings and wrapping the tortilla.

Cottage Cheese Delight: 5 minutes or less, depending on the toppings and mixing.

Breakfast Quiche Cups: 25-30 minutes, including preparation and baking time.

Breakfast Trail Mix: 5 minutes or less, depending on the ingredients and portioning.

Savory Oatmeal Bowl: 10-15 minutes, including cooking the oats and sautéing the vegetables.

Breakfast Quesadilla: 10-15 minutes, depending on the fillings and cooking time.

Green Smoothie Bowl: 5 minutes or less, depending on the blending and topping selection.

It's important to note that some recipes may require prepping ingredients in advance, such as soaking chia seeds overnight or cooking quinoa beforehand. Preparing ingredients ahead of time can significantly reduce the actual cooking time in the morning. Additionally, individual cooking skills and familiarity with the recipes can also impact the preparation time.

Make-ahead recipes for bars, muffins, and smoothie bowls

In today's fast-paced world, finding time for a nutritious breakfast can be a challenge. That's where make-ahead breakfast recipes come to the rescue. By preparing these delicious and wholesome breakfast bars, muffins, and smoothie bowls in advance, you can ensure a nourishing start to your day, even on the busiest of mornings.

Let's explore five mouthwatering recipes for each category that you can easily prepare and enjoy throughout the week.

<u>**Make-Ahead Breakfast Bars Recipes:**</u>
Almond Coconut Protein Bars:
Ingredients:
1 cup rolled oats
1 cup almond flour
1/2 cup unsweetened shredded coconut
1/4 cup protein powder (vanilla or your preferred flavor)
1/4 cup almond butter
1/4 cup honey or maple syrup
1/4 cup melted coconut oil
1/4 cup chopped almonds
1/4 cup dried cranberries or raisins
1 teaspoon vanilla extract
Pinch of salt
Preparation:

Preheat your oven to 350°F (175°C). Line a baking dish with parchment paper.

In a large mixing bowl, combine rolled oats, almond flour, shredded coconut, protein powder, chopped almonds, dried cranberries (or raisins), and salt.

In a separate microwave-safe bowl, heat the almond butter, honey (or maple syrup), and melted coconut oil together until smooth. You can microwave in short intervals, stirring in between, or melt on the stovetop over low heat.

Pour the almond butter mixture over the dry ingredients and mix well until all the ingredients are evenly combined and the mixture is slightly sticky.

Transfer the mixture into the prepared baking dish and press it down firmly using the back of a spoon or your hands.

Bake in the preheated oven for 15-20 minutes, or until the edges are golden brown.

Remove from the oven and let it cool completely in the baking dish. Once cooled, place it in the refrigerator for at least 2 hours to firm up.

Once chilled, lift the bars out of the baking dish using the parchment paper and cut them into desired-sized bars.

Blueberry Oat Bars:
Ingredients:
2 cups rolled oats
1 cup almond flour
1/2 cup almond butter
1/4 cup maple syrup
1/4 cup unsweetened applesauce
1 tsp vanilla extract
1 cup fresh blueberries
Preparation:

Preheat the oven to 350°F (175°C) and line a baking dish with parchment paper.

In a mixing bowl, combine oats, almond flour, almond butter, maple syrup, applesauce, and vanilla extract. Mix until well combined.

Gently fold in the fresh blueberries.

Transfer the mixture to the prepared baking dish and press it down evenly.

Bake for 25-30 minutes, or until the top turns golden brown.

Allow the bars to cool completely before cutting into individual servings.

Peanut Butter Chocolate Chip Bars:
Ingredients:

2 cups rolled oats
1 cup peanut butter
1/2 cup honey or maple syrup
1/4 cup unsweetened cocoa powder
1/4 cup chocolate chips
1 tsp vanilla extract
Preparation:

In a large mixing bowl, combine oats, peanut butter, honey (or maple syrup), cocoa powder, chocolate chips, and vanilla extract. Mix until all ingredients are well incorporated.

Transfer the mixture to a baking dish lined with parchment paper, pressing it down firmly.

Refrigerate for at least 2 hours, or until the bars are firm.

Once set, remove from the refrigerator and cut into desired-sized bars.

Almond Joy Breakfast Bars:
Ingredients:

1 1/2 cups almond flour
1/2 cup shredded coconut
1/4 cup almond butter
1/4 cup honey or maple syrup
1/4 cup melted coconut oil
1/4 cup dark chocolate chips
1/4 cup chopped almonds
Preparation:

In a mixing bowl, combine almond flour, shredded coconut, almond butter, honey (or maple syrup), and melted coconut oil. Stir until well combined.

Fold in the dark chocolate chips and chopped almonds.

Press the mixture into a baking dish lined with parchment paper, spreading it evenly.

Place in the refrigerator for at least 2 hours to allow the bars to set.

Once firm, cut into bars and store in an airtight container in the refrigerator.

Raspberry Quinoa Bars:
Ingredients:

1 1/2 cups cooked quinoa
1 cup almond flour
1/4 cup maple syrup

2 tbsp almond butter
1/4 cup unsweetened applesauce
1 cup fresh or frozen raspberries
1 tsp vanilla extract
Preparation:

Preheat the oven to 350°F (175°C) and line a baking dish with parchment paper.
In a mixing bowl, combine cooked quinoa, almond flour, maple syrup and almond butter. Mix well until the ingredients are thoroughly combined.
Add unsweetened applesauce and vanilla extract to the mixture and continue mixing until everything is evenly incorporated.
Gently fold in the fresh or frozen raspberries, being careful not to crush them too much.

Transfer the mixture to the prepared baking dish and spread it evenly, pressing it down firmly.
Bake in the preheated oven for 25-30 minutes, or until the edges are golden brown and the bars are set in the center. Remove from the oven and let the bars cool completely in the baking dish before cutting them into squares or rectangles.

Muffins Recipes:
Blueberry Lemon Chia Seed Muffins:

Ingredients:

2 cups all-purpose flour
1/2 cup granulated sugar
1 tablespoon baking powder
1/4 teaspoon salt
Zest of 1 lemon
3/4 cup unsweetened almond milk

1/4 cup lemon juice
1/4 cup melted coconut oil
2 tablespoons chia seeds
1 teaspoon vanilla extract
1 1/2 cups fresh or frozen blueberries
Preparation:

Preheat your oven to 375°F (190°C). Line a muffin tin with paper liners or grease it lightly.

In a large mixing bowl, whisk together the all-purpose flour, granulated sugar, baking powder, salt, and lemon zest.

In a separate bowl, combine the almond milk, lemon juice, melted coconut oil, chia seeds, and vanilla extract. Mix well.

Pour the wet ingredients into the dry ingredients and stir until just combined. Be careful not to overmix.

Gently fold in the blueberries, ensuring they are evenly distributed throughout the batter.

Divide the batter evenly among the muffin cups, filling each one about 3/4 full.

Bake for 18-22 minutes, or until a toothpick inserted into the center of a muffin comes out clean.

Allow the muffins to cool in the tin for 5 minutes, then transfer them to a wire rack to cool completely.

Banana Blueberry Walnut Muffins:
Ingredients:

2 cups all-purpose flour
1 teaspoon baking powder
1/2 teaspoon baking soda
1/4 teaspoon salt
1/2 teaspoon ground cinnamon

3 ripe bananas
1/2 cup almond milk
1 teaspoon vanilla extract
1 cup fresh or frozen blueberries
1/2 cup chopped walnuts
Preparation:

Preheat your oven to 350°F (175°C). Grease or line a muffin tin with paper liners.

In a large mixing bowl, whisk together the all-purpose flour, baking powder, baking soda, salt, and ground cinnamon. Set aside.

In a separate bowl, mash the bananas until smooth. Add the mashed bananas, almond milk, and vanilla extract to the dry ingredients. Mix well to combine.

Gently fold in the blueberries and chopped walnuts.

Spoon the batter into the prepared muffin tin, filling each cup about ¾ full.

Bake for 20-25 minutes, or until a toothpick inserted into the center of a muffin comes out clean.

Allow the muffins to cool in the tin for 5 minutes, then transfer them to a wire rack to cool completely.

Once cooled, store the muffins in an airtight container at room temperature for up to 3 days, or in the refrigerator for longer freshness.

Carrot Cake Muffins:
Ingredients:

2 cups whole wheat flour
1 ½ cups grated carrots
½ cup chopped walnuts
½ cup raisins
½ cup unsweetened applesauce

¼ cup coconut oil, melted
¼ cup maple syrup
2 tsp baking powder
1 tsp cinnamon
½ tsp nutmeg
¼ tsp salt
Preparation:

Preheat the oven to 350°F (175°C) and line a muffin tin with paper liners.
In a large mixing bowl, combine the whole wheat flour, grated carrots, chopped walnuts, and raisins.
In a separate bowl, whisk together the applesauce, melted coconut oil, maple syrup, baking powder, cinnamon, nutmeg, and salt.
Pour the wet ingredients into the dry ingredients and stir until just combined.

Divide the batter evenly among the muffin cups, filling each one about ¾ full.

Bake for 18-20 minutes, or until a toothpick inserted into the center of a muffin comes out clean.

Allow the muffins to cool in the tin for 5 minutes, then transfer them to a wire rack to cool completely.

Spinach and Feta Muffins:
Ingredients:

2 cups whole wheat flour
2 cups fresh spinach, chopped
1 cup crumbled feta cheese
½ cup chopped sun-dried tomatoes
½ cup chopped black olives
1 ¼ cups unsweetened almond milk
¼ cup olive oil
2 tsp baking powder
1 tsp dried oregano

½ tsp salt
Preparation:

Preheat the oven to 350°F (175°C) and line a muffin tin with paper liners.
In a large mixing bowl, combine the whole wheat flour, chopped spinach, crumbled feta cheese, chopped sun-dried tomatoes, and chopped black olives.
In a separate bowl, whisk together the almond milk, olive oil, baking powder, dried oregano, and salt.
Pour the wet ingredients into the dry ingredients and stir until just combined.
Divide the batter evenly among the muffin cups, filling each one about ¾ full.
Bake for 20-25 minutes, or until a toothpick inserted into the center of a muffin comes out clean.

Allow the muffins to cool in the tin for 5 minutes, then transfer them to a wire rack to cool completely.

Chocolate Zucchini Muffins:
Ingredients:

2 cups whole wheat flour
1 cup grated zucchini
½ cup cocoa powder
½ cup maple syrup
¼ cup coconut oil, melted
1 ¼ cups unsweetened almond milk
2 tsp baking powder
1 tsp vanilla extract
¼ tsp salt
Preparation:

Preheat the oven to 350°F (175°C) and line a muffin tin with paper liners.
In a large mixing bowl, combine the whole wheat flour, grated zucchini,

cocoa powder, maple syrup, melted coconut oil, almond milk, baking powder, vanilla extract, and salt. Stir until well combined.

Divide the batter evenly among the muffin cups, filling each one about ¾ full.

Optional: Sprinkle some chocolate chips on top of each muffin for extra indulgence.

Bake for 20-25 minutes, or until a toothpick inserted into the center of a muffin comes out clean.

Allow the muffins to cool in the tin for 5 minutes, then transfer them to a wire rack to cool completely.

Smoothie Bowl Recipes:
Berry Bliss Smoothie Bowl:
Ingredients:
1 cup frozen mixed berries (strawberries, blueberries, raspberries)
1 ripe banana
½ cup unsweetened almond milk
1 tbsp chia seeds
Toppings: sliced banana, fresh berries, granola, shredded coconut
Preparation:

In a blender, combine the frozen mixed berries, ripe banana, almond milk, and chia seeds. Blend until smooth and creamy.
Pour the smoothie into a bowl and add your desired toppings, such as sliced banana, fresh berries, granola, and shredded coconut.
Enjoy immediately.

Tropical Paradise Smoothie Bowl:

Ingredients:

1 cup frozen mango chunks
1 ripe banana
½ cup unsweetened coconut milk
1 tbsp shredded coconut
Toppings: sliced banana, chopped pineapple, kiwi slices, granola, hemp seeds
Preparation:

In a blender, combine the frozen mango chunks, ripe banana, coconut milk, and shredded coconut. Blend until smooth and creamy.
Pour the smoothie into a bowl and add your desired toppings, such as sliced banana, chopped pineapple, kiwi slices, granola, and hemp seeds.

Enjoy immediately.

Green Goddess Smoothie Bowl:

Ingredients:

1 cup fresh spinach
1 ripe banana
½ cup unsweetened almond milk
1 tbsp almond butter
Toppings: sliced banana, fresh berries, chia seeds, granola
Preparation:

In a blender, combine the fresh spinach, ripe banana, almond milk, and almond butter. Blend until smooth and creamy.
Pour the smoothie into a bowl and add your desired toppings, such as sliced banana, fresh berries, chia seeds, and granola.

Enjoy immediately.

Chocolate Peanut Butter Smoothie Bowl:

Ingredients:

1 ripe banana
2 tbsp unsweetened cocoa powder
2 tbsp peanut butter
½ cup unsweetened almond milk
Toppings: sliced banana, chopped peanuts, cacao nibs, shredded coconut
Preparation:

In a blender, combine the ripe banana, cocoa powder, peanut butter, and almond milk. Blend until smooth and creamy.
Pour the smoothie into a bowl and add your desired toppings, such as sliced

banana, chopped peanuts, cacao nibs, and shredded coconut.
Enjoy immediately.

Mixed Berry and Almond Smoothie Bowl:
Ingredients:

1 cup frozen mixed berries (strawberries, blueberries, raspberries)
1 ripe banana
½ cup unsweetened almond milk
2 tbsp almond butter
Toppings: sliced banana, fresh berries, almond slices, granola
Preparation:

In a blender, combine the frozen mixed berries, ripe banana, almond milk, and almond butter. Blend until smooth and creamy.

Pour the smoothie into a bowl and add your desired toppings, such as sliced banana, fresh berries, almond slices, and granola.
Enjoy immediately.

These make-ahead breakfast bars, muffins, and smoothie bowls provide delicious and convenient options to start your day on a nutritious note. By preparing these recipes in advance, you can ensure that you have a wholesome breakfast available even on the busiest of mornings. Enjoy the variety of flavors, textures, and nutrients that these recipes offer and embrace the ease and convenience of a delicious breakfast to kickstart your day.

Strategies for planning and prepping breakfasts in advance

Planning and prepping breakfasts in advance is a smart and effective way to ensure a healthy start to your day, especially for individuals with busy schedules. By dedicating some time to meal preparation, you can save valuable time in the mornings and make nutritious choices that align with your health goals. In this section, we will explore some strategies for planning and prepping breakfasts in advance.

Set aside time for meal planning: Dedicate a specific time each week to plan your breakfasts. Consider your schedule and choose recipes that are convenient and meet your nutritional needs. Look for recipes that can be prepared in advance, such as make-ahead breakfast bars, overnight oats, or smoothie freezer packs.

Create a weekly meal plan: Outline your breakfast options for the entire week. This will help you stay organized and ensure that you have all the necessary ingredients on hand. Consider incorporating a mix of recipes to keep your breakfasts interesting and varied.

Batch cook ingredients: Prep ingredients that can be used in multiple breakfast recipes. For example, cook a big batch of quinoa, chop vegetables, or make a large batch of homemade granola. Having these ingredients ready to go will make assembling breakfasts much quicker and easier.

Make use of overnight recipes: Overnight oats, chia seed puddings, and yogurt parfaits are great options for a quick and nutritious breakfast. Prepare them the night before and simply grab them from the refrigerator in the morning. These recipes often require minimal effort and can be customized with your favorite toppings and flavors.

Utilize freezer-friendly options: Prepare batches of muffins, breakfast burritos, or breakfast sandwiches and freeze them individually. In the morning, you can simply grab one from the freezer, heat it up, and enjoy a delicious and convenient breakfast in minutes.

Portion out ingredients: If you enjoy smoothies, pre-portion and freeze your favorite smoothie ingredients in individual bags or containers. This way, you can easily blend them in the morning without the need for measuring or chopping.

Invest in meal prep containers: Purchase a set of meal prep containers to store your prepped ingredients and meals. These containers are convenient for portioning out breakfasts and keeping them fresh. Consider using separate compartments for different ingredients or meals to maintain their flavors and textures.

Take advantage of slow cookers and instant pots: These kitchen appliances can be a time-saving solution for preparing breakfasts. Use your slow cooker to make overnight breakfast casseroles or set your instant pot to cook steel-cut oats for a warm and hearty breakfast.

Keep a well-stocked pantry: Make sure your pantry is stocked with essential breakfast ingredients such as oats, nuts, seeds, nut butter, whole-grain bread, and dried fruits. This will allow you to easily assemble quick and healthy breakfasts even on the busiest of mornings.

Stay organized and label your prepped meals: To avoid confusion and ensure freshness, label your prepped breakfasts with the date and contents.

This will help you keep track of what needs to be consumed first and maintain food safety.

By incorporating these strategies into your routine, you can enjoy a stress-free and nutritious breakfast every day. Planning and prepping in advance not only saves time but also helps you make mindful choices that align with your dietary goals.

Start experimenting with different recipes and find a meal prep routine that works best for you. With a little effort and organization, you can set yourself up for a healthy and successful start to the day.

1Week Meal plan you can consider

Here's a sample one-week meal plan that focuses on quick and healthy breakfasts while supporting weight loss goals and maintaining organization.

Day 1:

Overnight Chia Seed Pudding: Prepare the night before by mixing chia seeds, almond milk, and a sweetener of your choice. Top with fresh berries in the morning.

Day 2:

Make-Ahead Breakfast Burritos: Prepare a batch of breakfast burritos with whole-wheat tortillas, scrambled eggs or tofu, vegetables, and a sprinkle of cheese. Wrap them individually in foil and freeze. Reheat in the microwave in the morning.

Day 3:

Greek Yogurt Parfait: Layer Greek yogurt with homemade granola and a variety of fresh fruits. Prepare the granola in advance and store in an airtight container.

Day 4:

Veggie Egg Muffins: Make a batch of egg muffins filled with chopped vegetables and herbs. Bake them in advance and store in the refrigerator. Reheat in the morning for a protein-packed breakfast.

Day 5:

Green Smoothie Freezer Packs: Prepare individual freezer packs with pre-portioned ingredients for green smoothies. Include ingredients like spinach, kale, frozen fruits, and a source of plant-based protein. In the morning, simply blend the contents of the pack with water or almond milk.

Day 6:

Quinoa Breakfast Bowl: Cook a batch of quinoa and portion it into containers. In the morning, heat up the quinoa and top it with sliced bananas, almond butter, and a sprinkle of cinnamon.

<u>**Day 7:**</u>

Peanut Butter Banana Oatmeal Bars: Make a batch of homemade oatmeal bars using oats, mashed bananas, peanut butter, and a touch of sweetness like honey or maple syrup. Store them in an airtight container for grab-and-go breakfasts.

Remember to adapt the portion sizes according to your specific needs and consult with a healthcare professional or registered dietitian for personalized advice. Additionally, feel free to swap ingredients or recipes to suit your preferences and dietary restrictions. The key is to plan, prep, and organize your breakfasts in advance to support your weight loss goals and ensure a quick and healthy start to each day.

Chapter 8: The Science of Weight Loss: How Food Affects Your Body and Mind

In this chapter, we delve into the fascinating science behind weight loss and explore how the food we consume can profoundly impact our bodies and minds. By understanding the intricate relationship between food and weight management, we can make informed choices that support our health goals and create sustainable habits for long-term success.

The Role of Calories:
Calories play a crucial role in weight loss. We examine the concept of energy balance, where the calories we consume from food are compared to the calories we expend through daily activities and exercise. By creating a calorie deficit,

we encourage the body to tap into stored fat for energy, resulting in weight loss.

Macronutrients and Weight Loss:

We explore the importance of macronutrients—carbohydrates, proteins, and fats—in our diet and their impact on weight loss. Each macronutrient has a unique role in the body, affecting satiety, metabolism, and energy levels. We discuss how balancing macronutrient intake can optimize weight loss outcomes and provide practical strategies for incorporating them into meals.

The Role of Fiber:

Fiber is a key component of a weight loss-friendly diet. We delve into the science behind fiber's impact on satiety, digestion, and blood sugar regulation. By including fiber-rich foods like fruits, vegetables, whole grains, and legumes, we can enhance feelings of fullness, control cravings, and promote healthy weight management.

The Influence of Protein:
Protein is known for its role in building and repairing tissues, but it also plays a crucial role in weight loss. We explore the science behind protein's effect on satiety, thermogenesis, and muscle preservation. By including adequate protein in our meals, we can feel more satisfied, boost metabolism, and preserve lean muscle mass while losing weight.

The Impact of Carbohydrates:
Carbohydrates have often been scrutinized in weight loss discussions.

We delve into the different types of carbohydrates, such as complex carbs and simple sugars, and their effects on blood sugar, insulin levels, and energy. By choosing quality carbohydrates from whole grains, fruits, and vegetables, we can support sustainable weight loss while nourishing our bodies with essential nutrients.

The Role of Fats:
Fats have long been misunderstood in weight loss efforts. We explore the science behind healthy fats, such as monounsaturated and polyunsaturated fats, and their role in satiety, hormone regulation, and nutrient absorption. By incorporating sources of healthy fats, such as avocados, nuts, and olive oil, we can enhance the nutritional value of our meals and support weight loss.

The Psychology of Eating:
We delve into the psychological aspects of eating and their impact on weight management. We explore topics such as mindful eating, emotional eating, and food cravings. By developing a mindful and intuitive approach to eating, we can cultivate a healthier relationship with food and make choices that align with our weight loss goals.

Nutrition and Long-Term Weight Maintenance:
Finally, we discuss the importance of sustainable nutrition practices for long-term weight maintenance. We explore the role of balanced meals, portion control, and mindful indulgences in creating a healthy and enjoyable eating pattern that supports weight management. By adopting a holistic approach to nutrition, we can

achieve not only short-term weight loss but also long-term success in maintaining a healthy weight. Now let's delve deeper into the above mentioned topics in this chapter.

The Role of Calories: Understanding Energy Balance for Successful Weight Loss

When it comes to weight loss, understanding the role of calories is paramount. In this chapter, we will delve into the concept of energy balance, which forms the foundation for effective weight management.

By examining the relationship between the calories we consume and the calories we expend, we can gain valuable insights into how to achieve and maintain a healthy weight. So, let's explore the fascinating world of energy balance and its impact on our weight loss journey.

The Concept of Energy Balance:
Energy balance is the fundamental principle that governs weight regulation. It refers to the equilibrium between the calories we consume through food and beverages and the calories we expend through daily activities, exercise, and bodily functions. When energy intake matches energy expenditure, our weight remains stable. However, to lose weight, we need to create a calorie deficit by consuming fewer calories than we burn.

Calories In vs. Calories Out:
To effectively manage our weight, we must carefully consider the balance between calories in and calories out.

Calories represent the energy we obtain from the foods and beverages we consume. On the other hand, calories out include the energy expended through basal metabolic rate (BMR), physical activity, and the thermic effect of food (TEF).

Basal Metabolic Rate (BMR):
Basal metabolic rate (BMR) is the energy expended by our body at rest to maintain essential functions such as breathing, circulation, and cell production. It accounts for a significant portion of our daily calorie expenditure. Several factors influence our BMR, including age, gender, body composition, and genetics. Understanding our BMR helps us estimate our calorie needs and adjust our intake accordingly.

Physical Activity:
Physical activity plays a vital role in weight management. It encompasses any movement we engage in, from structured exercise sessions to everyday activities like walking, cleaning, or gardening. Increasing physical activity not only burns calories but also improves cardiovascular health, boosts metabolism, and enhances overall well-being. Finding enjoyable ways to incorporate more movement into our daily routine can contribute to sustained weight loss.

Thermic Effect of Food (TEF):
The thermic effect of food (TEF) refers to the energy required for digestion, absorption, and metabolism of nutrients. Different macronutrients have varying effects on TEF. For instance, protein requires more energy

to digest compared to carbohydrates or fats. By including protein-rich foods in our diet, we can slightly increase our calorie expenditure through the TEF, contributing to weight management.

Creating a Calorie Deficit:
To lose weight, we need to create a calorie deficit by consuming fewer calories than we burn. However, it is important to approach calorie reduction in a balanced and sustainable manner. Severely restricting calories can lead to nutrient deficiencies, decreased energy levels, and a slowdown in metabolism. Gradual and moderate calorie reduction, combined with increased physical activity, is a more sustainable approach to achieving and maintaining weight loss.

The Quality of Calories:
While calorie balance is crucial, the quality of calories also matters for overall health and well-being. Opting for nutrient-dense foods that provide essential vitamins, minerals, and fiber is vital for maintaining optimal health during the weight loss journey. Whole grains, lean proteins, fruits, vegetables, and healthy fats should form the basis of a balanced diet, ensuring that we meet our nutritional needs while managing our weight.

Understanding the role of calories and energy balance is essential for successful weight loss. By carefully considering the calories we consume and the calories we expend, we can create a sustainable calorie deficit that supports our weight loss goals. Striving for a balance between calorie intake, physical activity, and nutrient density allows us to achieve a healthy weight while nourishing our bodies with the essential nutrients they need. Remember, weight loss is a journey, and with a clear understanding of calories and energy balance, you can navigate this journey with confidence and achieve long-term success.

Macronutrients and Weight Loss: The Key to Balanced Nutrition and Optimal Results

In the journey towards weight loss, understanding the role of macronutrients is essential. Carbohydrates, proteins, and fats are the building blocks of our diet, each playing a distinct role in our body's functions. This article delves into the significance of macronutrients in relation to weight loss, exploring their effects on satiety, metabolism, and energy levels. We will also provide practical strategies for incorporating balanced macronutrients into our meals to optimize weight loss outcomes.

The Role of Carbohydrates:
Carbohydrates are the primary source of energy for our bodies. They provide glucose, which fuels our muscles and brain. However, not all carbohydrates are created equal. Complex carbohydrates, such as whole grains, fruits, and vegetables, are rich in fiber and nutrients, providing sustained energy and promoting satiety. On the other hand, refined carbohydrates, such as processed grains and sugars, can lead to rapid blood sugar spikes and crashes. By focusing on complex

carbohydrates and mindful portion control, we can harness their energy while promoting weight loss.

The Power of Proteins:
Proteins are the building blocks of our body's tissues, playing a crucial role in muscle repair and growth. Including adequate protein in our diet is essential for weight loss as it promotes satiety, helps preserve lean muscle mass, and supports a healthy metabolism. Lean sources of protein, such as poultry, fish, tofu, legumes, and low-fat dairy, can be incorporated into meals to provide a sense of fullness and aid in weight loss. Balancing protein intake throughout the day can also help regulate blood sugar levels and curb cravings.

Understanding Healthy Fats:
Fats are often misunderstood, but they play a vital role in our overall health and weight loss journey. Healthy fats, such as those found in avocados, nuts, seeds, and olive oil, provide essential fatty acids and fat-soluble vitamins. They contribute to satiety, help absorb nutrients, and support brain function.

Incorporating moderate amounts of healthy fats into our meals can promote long-term weight loss by keeping us satisfied and preventing overeating. It is important to avoid or limit unhealthy fats found in processed foods and deep-fried items, as they can hinder weight loss efforts.

Achieving Macronutrient Balance:
Optimizing weight loss outcomes involves achieving a balanced intake of macronutrients. This can be achieved by focusing on portion control, mindful eating, and meal planning. Start by including a variety of colorful fruits and vegetables to increase fiber and nutrient intake.

Pair complex carbohydrates with lean proteins to enhance satiety and control blood sugar levels. Incorporate healthy fats in moderation to add flavor and support overall health. By planning meals that include all macronutrients in balanced proportions, we can create a sustainable approach to weight loss.

Practical Strategies for Incorporating Macronutrients:

To effectively incorporate macronutrients into our meals, it is helpful to plan ahead and diversify our food choices. Consider batch cooking and meal prepping to ensure a well-balanced and time-efficient approach. Experiment with different recipes that incorporate a variety of macronutrients, such as grain bowls with roasted vegetables, lean protein salads, and plant-based stir-fries. Pay attention to portion sizes and listen to your body's hunger and fullness cues.

Seek guidance from a registered dietitian or nutritionist to personalize your macronutrient intake based on your specific needs and weight loss goals. Understanding the role of macronutrients in weight loss is crucial for achieving balanced nutrition and optimal results. By incorporating complex carbohydrates, lean proteins, and healthy fats in our meals, we can harness the benefits of each macronutrient to support satiety, metabolism, and overall well-being. Balancing macronutrients and adopting mindful eating practices can create a sustainable approach to weight loss that promotes long-term success.

Remember, consulting with a healthcare professional or registered dietitian can provide personalized guidance and support on your journey towards achieving your weight loss goals.

The Role of Fiber in Weight Loss: A Science-Based Approach to Satiety and Digestive Health

When it comes to weight loss, incorporating fiber into our diet is a smart strategy. Fiber offers numerous health benefits, including improved digestion, enhanced satiety, and better blood sugar regulation. In this article, we will delve into the science behind fiber's impact on weight loss and explore how it can be integrated into our daily eating habits for optimal results.

Understanding Fiber:

Fiber is a type of carbohydrate found in plant-based foods, such as fruits, vegetables, whole grains, legumes, and nuts. Unlike other carbohydrates, fiber cannot be fully digested by the body, so it passes through our digestive system relatively intact. There are two main types of fiber: soluble fiber, which dissolves in water, and insoluble fiber, which does not dissolve. Both types of fiber contribute to our overall health and play a vital role in weight management.

The Impact of Fiber on Satiety:
One of the key benefits of fiber is its ability to promote satiety, the feeling of fullness after a meal. When we consume high-fiber foods, they take longer to digest, slowing down the emptying of the stomach and increasing the time it takes for nutrients to be absorbed. This prolonged digestion process can help us feel satisfied for longer periods, reducing the likelihood of overeating or snacking between meals. Including fiber-rich foods in our breakfast can set the tone for the rest of the day, keeping

hunger at bay and supporting our weight loss goals.

The Influence of Fiber on Digestive Health:

Fiber plays a crucial role in maintaining a healthy digestive system. Soluble fiber absorbs water in the intestines, forming a gel-like substance that softens the stool and promotes regular bowel movements. Insoluble fiber, on the other hand, adds bulk to the stool, facilitating its movement through the digestive tract. A healthy and efficient digestive system is essential for weight loss, as it helps eliminate waste and toxins from the body, preventing bloating and discomfort. By incorporating fiber-rich foods, we can support optimal digestive health and create a foundation for successful weight management.

Blood Sugar Regulation and Fiber:
Fiber has a significant impact on blood sugar regulation. Soluble fiber slows down the absorption of glucose into the bloodstream, preventing rapid spikes in blood sugar levels. This steady release of glucose helps to stabilize energy levels and prevent cravings for sugary foods. By incorporating fiber-rich carbohydrates into our meals, such as whole grains and legumes, we can achieve more balanced blood sugar levels, supporting weight loss efforts and overall metabolic health.

Practical Strategies for Increasing Fiber Intake:
To boost fiber intake, it is important to include a variety of plant-based foods in our diet. Start by incorporating more fruits, vegetables, and whole grains

into meals and snacks. Experiment with new recipes that feature fiber-rich ingredients, such as roasted vegetable quinoa bowls, lentil soups, or chia seed puddings. Gradually increase fiber intake to allow your body to adjust and avoid digestive discomfort. Remember to drink plenty of water throughout the day, as fiber works best when combined with adequate hydration.

Fiber plays a crucial role in weight loss by promoting satiety, supporting digestive health, and regulating blood sugar levels. By incorporating fiber-rich foods into our daily eating habits, we can harness these benefits and create a solid foundation for achieving and maintaining a healthy weight. Aim to consume a diverse range of plant-based foods and gradually increase your fiber intake to optimize weight loss outcomes. As always, consult with a healthcare professional or registered dietitian to tailor your fiber intake to your specific needs and goals.

The Influence of Protein on Weight Loss: Unveiling the Science Behind Satiety, Thermogenesis, and Muscle Preservation

Protein is often hailed as the building block of life, essential for muscle growth and repair. However, its benefits extend far beyond that. Protein also plays a critical role in weight loss, thanks to its effects on satiety, thermogenesis, and muscle preservation. In this article, we will delve into the science behind protein's influence on weight management and explore how incorporating adequate protein into our diet can enhance our weight loss journey.

Understanding Protein:
Protein is a macronutrient made up of amino acids, which are the building blocks of our body's tissues, including muscles, organs, and skin. When we consume protein-rich foods, our body breaks them down into amino acids, which are then utilized for various physiological functions. Protein can be found in both animal-based sources, such as meat, poultry, fish, and dairy, as well as plant-based sources like legumes, tofu, tempeh, and quinoa.

Satiety and Protein:

One of the key benefits of protein for weight loss is its impact on satiety—the feeling of fullness after a meal. Protein is known to be more filling than carbohydrates or fats due to its effect on appetite-regulating hormones, such as ghrelin and peptide YY. Consuming protein-rich foods can help curb hunger and reduce the likelihood of overeating or snacking between meals. By prioritizing protein at breakfast, we set the stage for a day of controlled food intake, aiding in weight loss efforts.

Thermogenesis and Protein:

Thermogenesis refers to the energy expenditure that occurs during the digestion, absorption, and processing of food. Protein has a higher thermic effect compared to carbohydrates and fats, meaning that our body burns more calories during the digestion of protein-rich foods. This increased energy expenditure can contribute to weight loss by boosting our metabolism and supporting a calorie deficit. Incorporating protein into our meals can help maximize the thermic effect, aiding in our weight loss goals.

Muscle Preservation and Protein:
During weight loss, it is crucial to preserve lean muscle mass, as it contributes to a higher metabolic rate and overall body composition. Protein plays a pivotal role in muscle preservation. Adequate protein intake provides the essential amino acids needed for muscle protein synthesis, which helps repair and build new muscle tissue. By ensuring sufficient protein intake, we can promote muscle

preservation and mitigate the risk of muscle loss during weight loss efforts.

Practical Strategies for Incorporating Protein:

To optimize the benefits of protein for weight loss, it is important to incorporate protein-rich foods into each meal and snack. Aim to include lean sources of protein, such as skinless chicken, turkey, fish, eggs, tofu, Greek yogurt, and legumes. Distribute your protein intake evenly throughout the day to support muscle protein synthesis and maintain satiety.

Experiment with recipes that combine protein with fiber-rich vegetables and whole grains for a well-rounded, satisfying meal.

Protein's influence on weight loss extends beyond its role in muscle growth and repair. It also impacts satiety, thermogenesis, and muscle preservation. By incorporating protein-rich foods into our diet and distributing protein intake throughout the day, we can enhance our weight loss efforts.

Remember to consult with a healthcare professional or registered dietitian to determine the appropriate protein intake for your individual needs and goals. Harness the power of protein to support your weight loss journey and achieve long-term success.

The Impact of Carbohydrates: Unraveling the Effects on Blood Sugar, Insulin Levels, and Energy

Carbohydrates are a fundamental macronutrient in our diet, providing us with energy to fuel our daily activities. However, not all carbohydrates are created equal. Different types of carbohydrates, such as complex carbs and simple sugars, have varying effects on our blood sugar levels, insulin response, and overall energy levels. In this article, we will delve into the impact of carbohydrates on weight management and explore how making informed choices about the types of carbohydrates we consume can positively influence our health and weight loss goals.

Understanding Carbohydrates:
Carbohydrates are compounds made up of sugar molecules, which are the body's primary source of energy. They can be classified into two main categories: complex carbohydrates and simple sugars. Complex carbohydrates, found in whole grains, legumes, and vegetables, consist of longer chains of sugar molecules and are digested and absorbed more slowly. Simple sugars, found in sweets, sugary beverages, and processed foods, are composed of shorter sugar chains and are quickly digested, leading to a rapid increase in blood sugar levels.

Blood Sugar and Carbohydrates:
When we consume carbohydrates, they are broken down into glucose, which enters our bloodstream and provides energy to our cells. The speed at which

this happens depends on the type of carbohydrates we consume. Complex carbohydrates, due to their longer chains, are digested more slowly, resulting in a gradual and steady rise in blood sugar levels. On the other hand, simple sugars are rapidly digested, leading to a sudden spike in blood sugar levels. This spike is followed by a rapid drop in blood sugar, which can leave us feeling fatigued and craving more carbohydrates.

Insulin Response and Carbohydrates:
Insulin is a hormone produced by the pancreas that plays a crucial role in regulating blood sugar levels. When blood sugar rises after a meal, insulin is released to help transport glucose into our cells for energy or storage. The type and amount of carbohydrates we consume can impact our insulin

response. Simple sugars cause a more significant and rapid release of insulin, which can lead to insulin spikes and potentially contribute to insulin resistance over time. Complex carbohydrates, on the other hand, result in a more controlled insulin response.

Energy and Carbohydrates:
Carbohydrates are our body's preferred source of energy, providing us with the fuel we need for physical activity and brain function. However, the type of carbohydrates we choose can affect our energy levels. Simple sugars, while providing a quick burst of energy, are often followed by a crash as blood sugar levels plummet. This can lead to feelings of fatigue and sluggishness. Complex carbohydrates, with their slower digestion and steady release of

glucose, provide sustained energy and help maintain stable energy levels throughout the day.

Making Informed Choices:
To optimize the impact of carbohydrates on weight management and overall health, it is essential to make informed choices about the types of carbohydrates we consume. Focus on incorporating more complex carbohydrates into your diet, such as whole grains, legumes, fruits, and vegetables. These provide a rich source of fiber, vitamins, and minerals while promoting stable blood sugar levels and sustained energy. Limit the consumption of simple sugars and processed foods, which can lead to blood sugar spikes, energy crashes, and contribute to weight gain.

Carbohydrates play a vital role in our diet, providing us with the energy we need for daily activities. By understanding the impact of carbohydrates on blood sugar, insulin levels, and energy, we can make informed choices that support our weight management goals and overall well-being.

Opt for complex carbohydrates that promote stable blood sugar levels and sustained energy, while limiting the intake of simple sugars and processed foods. Remember, balance and moderation are key when it comes to carbohydrates, ensuring a healthy and sustainable approach to weight loss and overall health.

The Role of Fats: Unlocking the Power of Healthy Fats for Satiety, Hormone Regulation, and Nutrient Absorption

For many years, fats were demonized as the enemy of weight loss and overall health. However, research has shown that not all fats are created equal. Healthy fats, such as monounsaturated and polyunsaturated fats, play a crucial role in our diet and can support our weight loss goals when consumed in moderation.

We will explore the science behind healthy fats and their impact on satiety, hormone regulation, and nutrient absorption, helping us make informed choices for optimal health and weight management.

Understanding Healthy Fats:
Healthy fats are a type of dietary fat that provides numerous health benefits when consumed in appropriate amounts. They are found in foods such as avocados, nuts, seeds, olive oil, fatty fish, and plant-based oils like flaxseed and walnut oil. These fats are known for their composition of monounsaturated and polyunsaturated fatty acids, which are considered beneficial for our health.

Satiety and Healthy Fats:
One of the remarkable properties of healthy fats is their ability to promote satiety, or the feeling of fullness and satisfaction after a meal. When we consume foods rich in healthy fats, they take longer to digest, allowing us to feel satisfied for a more extended

period. This can help prevent overeating and snacking between meals, supporting our weight loss efforts by reducing overall calorie intake.

Hormone Regulation and Healthy Fats: Healthy fats play a vital role in hormone regulation, including the production and balance of hormones involved in weight management. Certain hormones, such as leptin and ghrelin, are responsible for signaling hunger and fullness to our brain. Healthy fats can help regulate the production and sensitivity of these hormones, helping us maintain a healthy appetite and prevent overeating.

Nutrient Absorption and Healthy Fats:
Some vitamins and minerals are fat-soluble, which means they require the presence of dietary fats to be properly absorbed and utilized by our bodies. Vitamins A, D, E, and K are examples of fat-soluble vitamins. Consuming healthy fats alongside foods rich in these nutrients enhances their absorption and ensures we receive their full benefits. Additionally, healthy fats can enhance the flavors and textures of meals, making them more enjoyable and satisfying.

Incorporating Healthy Fats into Your Diet:
To harness the benefits of healthy fats for weight management and overall health, it is important to incorporate them into our daily diet. Opt for foods such as avocados, nuts, seeds, and fatty

fish like salmon and mackerel. Replace saturated and trans fats, found in processed foods and fried items, with healthier alternatives like olive oil or avocado oil for cooking and dressing. Aim for a balanced intake of healthy fats as part of a well-rounded diet, alongside other essential macronutrients.

Healthy fats, such as monounsaturated and polyunsaturated fats, are essential for our overall health and weight management. By understanding their role in promoting satiety, regulating hormones, and facilitating nutrient absorption, we can make informed choices to incorporate healthy fats into our diet. Opt for foods rich in healthy fats and use them as a replacement for unhealthy fats in cooking and meal preparation. Remember to practice moderation and balance in your overall diet, ensuring a healthy and sustainable approach to weight loss and overall well-being.

The Psychology of Eating: Understanding the Mind-Body Connection for Effective Weight Management

When it comes to weight management, it's not just about the food we eat, but also the psychological factors that influence our eating behaviors. The psychology of eating explores the intricate relationship between our mind and body when it comes to food choices, portion sizes, and overall eating patterns. In this article, we will delve into the psychological aspects of eating and their impact on weight management, focusing on mindful eating, emotional eating, and food cravings. By understanding these factors, we can develop a healthier relationship with food and achieve more effective weight management outcomes.

Mindful Eating:

The Power of Awareness:
Mindful eating is a practice that involves paying attention to our eating experience with non-judgmental awareness. By being fully present in the moment, we can cultivate a deeper connection with our food, our body, and our hunger and fullness cues. Mindful eating allows us to savor the flavors, textures, and aromas of our food, helping us make conscious choices and enjoy our meals without distractions. Research suggests that practicing mindful eating can lead to

healthier food choices, improved portion control, and enhanced overall satisfaction with meals, all of which can support weight management efforts.

Emotional Eating:

Understanding and Addressing Emotional Triggers:

Emotional eating refers to the tendency to use food as a way to cope with or soothe negative emotions such as stress, sadness, or boredom. Many individuals turn to food for comfort, seeking temporary relief from emotional discomfort. However, emotional eating can contribute to weight gain and hinder weight loss efforts. Understanding the underlying emotional triggers that lead to emotional eating is crucial for effective weight management. By identifying alternative coping strategies, such as engaging in physical activity, practicing relaxation techniques, or seeking support from loved ones, we can break the cycle of emotional eating and develop healthier ways to deal with our emotions.

Food Cravings:

Unraveling the Mystery:
Food cravings are intense desires for specific types of food, often high in sugar, fat, or salt. These cravings can feel overpowering and can lead to overeating or unhealthy food choices. Understanding the psychology behind food cravings can help us manage them more effectively. Cravings can be triggered by various factors, including emotional states, environmental cues,

and even hormonal fluctuations. By being aware of our triggers and finding healthier alternatives or ways to satisfy our cravings, such as opting for a small portion of the desired food or finding nutritious substitutes, we can regain control over our eating behaviors and support our weight management goals.

Developing a Healthy Relationship with Food:

To harness the power of the psychology of eating for weight management, it's important to develop a healthy relationship with food. This involves cultivating self-awareness, practicing mindfulness, and addressing emotional triggers in a constructive manner. By building a positive and balanced mindset around food, we can make nourishing choices that support our overall health and well-being. Seeking guidance from a qualified healthcare professional, such as a registered dietitian or therapist specializing in eating behaviors, can provide valuable support and strategies for developing a healthy relationship with food.

The psychology of eating plays a significant role in weight management, influencing our food choices, portion sizes, and overall eating behaviors. By understanding the concepts of mindful eating, emotional eating, and food cravings, we can develop a deeper awareness of our relationship with food and make conscious choices that support our weight management goals. By addressing emotional triggers, practicing mindfulness, and seeking professional guidance, we can establish a healthy mindset around food and achieve long-term success in maintaining a balanced and nourishing lifestyle.

Nutrition and Long-Term Weight Maintenance: Building Sustainable Habits for Lasting Success

Achieving weight loss is a significant accomplishment, but maintaining that weight loss over the long term requires a different approach. Sustainable nutrition practices play a crucial role in supporting lasting weight maintenance. In this article, we will explore the importance of balanced meals, portion control, and mindful indulgences in creating a healthy and enjoyable eating pattern that supports weight management. By adopting these practices, individuals can establish a sustainable and nourishing lifestyle that promotes long-term weight maintenance.

Balanced Meals: Nourishing Your Body for Sustained Success
Achieving and maintaining weight loss involves providing your body with the nutrients it needs while maintaining a calorie balance. Balanced meals, consisting of a combination of macronutrients (carbohydrates, proteins, and fats) along with an array of micronutrients (vitamins and minerals), are essential for supporting overall health and satiety. Including a variety of colorful fruits and vegetables, whole grains, lean proteins, and healthy fats in your meals ensures that your body receives the necessary nutrients for optimal function. Balanced meals not only provide sustained energy but also help control

cravings and maintain a healthy weight.

Portion Control: Finding the Right Balance.

Portion control is a key component of long-term weight maintenance. It involves being mindful of serving sizes and understanding the appropriate amounts of food to consume. Portion control allows individuals to manage their calorie intake effectively without feeling deprived. Strategies such as using smaller plates and bowls, measuring food portions, and practicing mindful eating can help maintain portion control. By being aware of portion sizes and practicing moderation, individuals can enjoy a wide variety of foods while still maintaining a healthy weight.

Mindful Indulgences: Enjoying Treats Without Guilt.
Depriving oneself of favorite foods can often lead to feelings of frustration and may result in unsustainable eating patterns. Mindful indulgences involve enjoying occasional treats while being mindful of portion sizes and the overall balance of one's diet. By savoring and fully experiencing indulgent foods, individuals can satisfy their cravings and prevent feelings of restriction.

Incorporating mindful indulgences into a balanced eating pattern promotes a positive relationship with food and helps maintain long-term weight management.

Sustainability and Consistency: The Key to Long-Term Success

Maintaining a healthy weight is not just about short-term changes but also about adopting sustainable habits. Consistency is crucial in establishing a routine that supports long-term weight maintenance.

This involves consistently practicing portion control, making balanced meal choices, and incorporating mindful indulgences into one's eating pattern. Building sustainable habits, such as meal planning, grocery shopping with a list, and finding enjoyable physical activities, helps create a lifestyle that supports ongoing weight management efforts.

Sustainable nutrition practices are essential for long-term weight maintenance. By focusing on balanced meals, portion control, and mindful indulgences, individuals can create a healthy and enjoyable eating pattern that supports weight management goals. Consistency and sustainability are key, as they enable individuals to establish lasting habits that promote overall health and well-being.

By embracing these practices and seeking support from healthcare professionals, individuals can achieve long-term success in maintaining a healthy weight and living a fulfilling and nourishing life.

Food and Mental Health

Food not only influences our physical health but also our mental well-being. Eating a diet that is rich in nutrient-dense foods may boost mood, decrease stress and anxiety, and improve general mental well-being. On the other side, a diet heavy in processed foods and added sugars may lead to sadness, anxiety, and other mental health disorders. Food and mental health are tightly related, and what we eat may have a big influence on our mood, stress levels, and general well-being. Eating a diet that is rich in nutrient-dense foods, such as fruits, vegetables, whole grains, lean proteins, and healthy fats, may give the body the critical elements it needs to operate correctly.

These nutrients, such as vitamins, minerals, and antioxidants, may promote the functioning of the brain and the nervous system, which can have a favorable influence on mental health. Eating a balanced diet that is rich in these nutrients may help enhance mood, decrease stress and anxiety, and improve general mental well-being. On the other side, a diet heavy in processed foods and added sugars may lead to sadness, anxiety, and other mental health disorders. These meals are frequently heavy in calories and poor in nutrients, which may contribute to weight gain, inflammation, and a number of other health concerns. Processed foods are also heavy in added sugars, which may cause blood sugar changes and contribute to mood swings and irritation.

The gut-brain axis, the communication network between the stomach and the brain, is also vital to examine when we speak about the link between food and mental health. The gut is home to trillions of bacteria, collectively known as gut microbiome, that play a crucial role in the digestion and absorption of nutrients, as well as in the control of the immune system and the neurological system. Research has revealed that the gut microbiota may impact our mental health, and an imbalance in the gut microbiome can lead to mental health concerns such as melancholy and anxiety. A diet that is strong in fiber, fermented foods, and probiotics may assist to sustain a healthy gut microbiota and boost mental well-being.

A diet that is rich in nutrient-dense foods, and balanced macronutrients that promote a healthy gut flora may have a good influence on mental health and well-being. Eating a balanced breakfast every day, with a combination of protein, healthy fats, and complex carbs may help set the tone for the rest of the day, keeping you full and content, with constant energy levels and a happy mood. We have covered the significance of nutrition in weight reduction, the relevance of macronutrients, and how various meals may affect our general health and well-being. It's vital to remember that weight reduction is not about restriction or deprivation but about building a sustainable and balanced diet that supplies your body with the energy and nutrition it needs.

Conclusion

Recap of key takeaways

In this book, we have explored various aspects of breakfast and its significance in achieving optimal health, weight management, and overall well-being. From understanding the importance of a nutritious breakfast to exploring creative and delicious recipes, we have covered a wide range of topics to empower you in making informed choices for your morning meals.

Starting with the benefits of breakfast, we highlighted how a well-balanced morning meal provides essential nutrients, supports cognitive function, and sets the tone for the day ahead. By incorporating a variety of ingredients such as fruits, whole grains, proteins, and healthy fats, trusting that you have gained insights into creating nourishing and satisfying breakfast options. We delved into the world of smoothies, showcasing their versatility and ability to pack a nutritional punch. From energy-boosting fruit-based smoothies to nutrient-rich green smoothies, with no doubt I know you have discovered a plethora of options to start your day on a vibrant note.

The chapter on wholesome cereal and oatmeal delights showcased the beauty of grains and their role in providing fiber, vitamins, and minerals. Through creative and nutritious recipes, readers have learned how to turn humble grains into delightful breakfast creations that are both wholesome and delicious.

Eggs, as a protein powerhouse, took center stage in our exploration of protein-packed breakfasts. From omelets and frittatas to egg muffins, am sure you have discovered numerous ways to incorporate eggs into your morning routine, whether you're following a vegetarian or vegan lifestyle.

The power of plant-based breakfasts emerged as a significant theme, highlighting the growing popularity and benefits of plant-based diets. With a focus on nutrient-dense ingredients, readers have been introduced to a variety of plant-based breakfast options that provide nourishment from nature. We also acknowledged the need for quick and convenient breakfast options for busy individuals, offering ideas for grab-and-go meals that can be prepared in advance. With recipes for make-ahead breakfast bars, muffins, and smoothie bowls, we are convinced that you have gained inspiration for satisfying meals that can be enjoyed even on the busiest of mornings.

Finally, we delved into the science of weight loss and explored the impact of food on the body and mind. By understanding the role of calories, macronutrients, fiber, protein, carbohydrates, and fats, readers have gained valuable insights into the science behind weight management and how to make informed dietary choices. Throughout this book, our aim has been to provide you with a comprehensive guide to creating nourishing, delicious, and satisfying breakfasts that support their health goals. Whether one seeks to boost energy, achieve weight loss, or simply start the day on a positive note, the recipes, strategies, and knowledge shared in this book are designed to inspire and empower you on your breakfast journey.

Remember, breakfast is not just a meal; it's an opportunity to nourish the body, invigorate the mind, and set the stage for a vibrant and fulfilling day. Embrace the power of breakfast and make it a delightful and nourishing part of your daily routine.

Encouragement to experiment with recipes and tips

In closing, I want to encourage you to embrace the spirit of experimentation and exploration when it comes to breakfast. The recipes and ideas presented in this book are just the beginning of your breakfast journey. Don't be afraid to get creative in the kitchen and customize recipes to suit your taste preferences and dietary needs.

Try swapping out ingredients, adding new flavors and textures, and experimenting with different cooking methods. Breakfast should never be boring, so let your imagination run wild and discover new favorite combinations that bring excitement to your mornings. Additionally, I encourage you to take advantage of the tips and strategies shared throughout this book. Planning and prepping your breakfasts in advance can save you time and ensure that you have nutritious options readily available, even on hectic mornings. Incorporating a balance of macronutrients, fiber, and protein in your breakfasts can help you feel satisfied and energized throughout the day.

Remember, breakfast is a chance to nourish your body and set a positive tone for the day. It's an opportunity to savor delicious flavors, explore new ingredients, and prioritize your well-being. So, be adventurous, have fun in the kitchen, and enjoy the journey of creating nutritious and satisfying breakfasts that support your health and wellness goals. Wishing you a delightful breakfast experience filled with nourishment, creativity, and enjoyment. Cheers to a vibrant and fulfilling start to your day! Am Dora Feest.

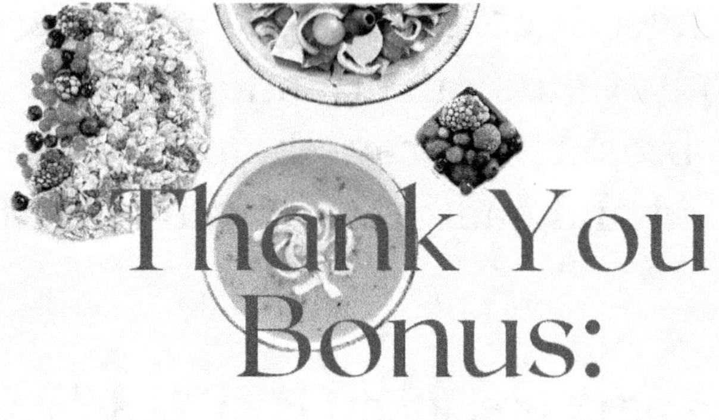

Thank You & Bonus:

2 Month Meal Plan

The following is a two month meal plan for weight loss. It includes a balance of carbohydrates, protein, and healthy fats, as well as a variety of fruits and vegetables. It also includes options for breakfast, lunch, and dinner, as well as snacks.

Dora Feest

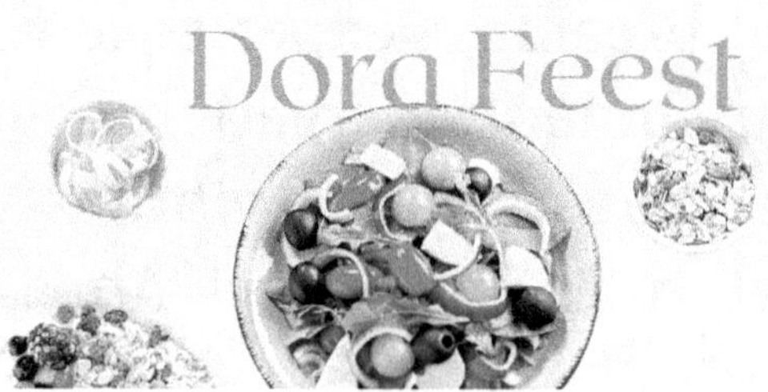

Thank You Bonus:

Here's Our Thank You Bonus For Buying This Book Meal Plan for Two Months of Weight Loss

Week 1:

Day 1:

Breakfast: Greek yogurt with berries and a sprinkle of granola

Snack: Apple slices with almond butter

Lunch: Grilled chicken breast with roasted vegetables and quinoa

Snack: Celery sticks with hummus

Dinner: Baked salmon with a side salad

Day 2:

Breakfast: Oatmeal with banana slices and a drizzle of honey

Snack: Carrots and cucumber slices with tzatziki dip

Lunch: Turkey and avocado wrap with a side of fruit

Snack: Greek yogurt with honey and a sprinkle of chia seeds

Dinner: Stir-fry with chicken, vegetables, and brown rice

Day 3:

Breakfast: Scrambled eggs with spinach and mushrooms

Snack: Berries and low-fat cottage cheese

Lunch: Grilled chicken Caesar salad

Snack: Hard-boiled eggs

Dinner: Turkey chili with a side of roasted sweet potatoes

Day 4:

Breakfast: Smoothie bowl with Greek yogurt, berries, and spinach

Snack: Celery sticks with peanut butter

Lunch: Grilled fish with a side of roasted vegetables

Snack: Apple slices with cinnamon

Dinner: Baked chicken breast with a side of quinoa and steamed vegetables

Day 5:

Breakfast: Omelette with bell peppers, onions, and mushrooms

Snack: Berries and low-fat Greek yogurt

Lunch: Turkey burger with a side of roasted sweet potatoes

Snack: Carrots and cucumber slices with hummus

Dinner: Grilled shrimp with a side of quinoa and steamed vegetables

Day 6:

Breakfast: Scrambled eggs with spinach and tomatoes

Snack: Berries and low-fat cottage cheese

Lunch: Grilled chicken with a side of quinoa and steamed vegetables

Snack: Greek yogurt with honey and a sprinkle of chia seeds

Dinner: Baked salmon with a side of roasted vegetables

Day 7:

Breakfast: Smoothie bowl with Greek yogurt, berries, and spinach

Snack: Apple slices with almond butter

Lunch: Grilled fish with a side of roasted vegetables

Snack: Carrots and cucumber slices with tzatziki dip

Dinner: Stir-fry with chicken, vegetables, and brown rice

Week 2-8:

Repeat the same meal plan as week 1, but switch up the proteins and vegetables to add variety and prevent boredom.

Week 9-10:

Breakfast: Greek yogurt with berries and a sprinkle of granola

Snack: Apple slices with almond butter
Lunch: Grilled chicken breast with roasted vegetables and quinoa
Snack: Celery sticks with hummus
Dinner: Baked salmon with a side salad

Week 11-12:
Breakfast: Oatmeal with banana slices and a drizzle of honey
Snack: Carrots and cucumber slices with tzatziki dip

Lunch: Turkey and avocado wrap with a side of fruit
Snack: Greek yogurt with honey and a sprinkle of chia seeds
Dinner: Stir-fry with chicken, vegetables, and brown rice

Week 13-14:
Breakfast: Scrambled eggs with spinach and mushrooms

Snack: Berries and low-fat cottage cheese
Lunch: Grilled chicken Caesar salad
Snack: Hard-boiled eggs
Dinner: Turkey chili with a side of roasted sweet potatoes

Week 15-16:
Breakfast: Smoothie bowl with Greek yogurt, berries, and spinach
Snack: Celery sticks with peanut butter
Lunch: Grilled fish with a side of roasted vegetables
Snack: Apple slices with cinnamon
Dinner: Baked chicken breast with a side of quinoa and steamed vegetables

Week 17-18:
Breakfast: Omelette with bell peppers, onions, and mushrooms
Snack: Berries and low-fat Greek yogurt

Lunch: Turkey burger with a side of roasted sweet potatoes

Snack: Carrots and cucumber slices with hummus

Dinner: Grilled shrimp with a side of quinoa and steamed vegetables

Week 19-20:

Breakfast: Scrambled eggs with spinach and tomatoes

Snack: Berries and low-fat cottage cheese

Lunch: Grilled chicken with a side of quinoa and steamed vegetables

Snack: Greek yogurt with honey and a sprinkle of chia seeds

Dinner: Baked salmon with a side of roasted vegetables

Week 21-22:

Breakfast: Smoothie bowl with Greek yogurt, berries, and spinach

Snack: Apple slices with almond butter
Lunch: Grilled fish with a side of roasted vegetables
Snack: Carrots and cucumber slices with tzatziki dip
Dinner: Stir-fry with chicken, vegetables, and brown rice

<u>**Week 23-24:**</u>
Breakfast: Greek yogurt with berries and a sprinkle of granola
Snack: Apple slices with almond butter
Lunch: Grilled chicken breast with roasted vegetables and quinoa
Snack: Celery sticks with hummus
Dinner: Baked salmon with a side salad

Note: *This meal plan is designed for a person who is trying to lose weight and should be adjusted based on individual calorie needs. It is important to also incorporate regular physical activity and consult with a healthcare professional before making any drastic changes to your diet.*